DR. SPOCK'S PREGNANCY GUIDE

There are many popular pregnancy guides available, but only one that offers parents-to-be the knowledge and experience of the trusted experts at The Dr. Spock Company. In one handy reference, you'll discover all you need to know about:

Dealing with pregnancy symptoms

Understanding your body's changes

Getting the best care available

Preparing for labor and delivery

And much more!

D0440361

BOOKS BY BENJAMIN SPOCK, M.D.

Dr. Spock's Baby and Child Care

Dr. Spock on Parenting

Dr. Spock's The First Two Years

Dr. Spock's The School Years

BOOKS FROM THE DR. SPOCK COMPANY

Take Charge Parenting Guides:

Dr. Spock's Baby Basics

Dr. Spock's Pregnancy Guide

Published by POCKET BOOKS

DR. SPOCK'S
PREGNANCY GUIDE

MARJORIE GREENFIELD, M.D.

POCKET BOOKS

New York   London   Toronto   Sydney   Singapore

The ideas, procedures and suggestions in this book are intended to supplement,
not replace, the medical advice of trained professionals. All matters regarding
your health require medical supervision. Consult your physician before adopting
the medical suggestions in this book as well as about any condition that may
require diagnosis or medical attention. The authors and publisher disclaim any
liability arising directly or indirectly from the use of this book.

An *Original* Publication of POCKET BOOKS

POCKET BOOKS, a division of Simon & Schuster, Inc.
1230 Avenue of the Americas, New York, NY 10020

ISBN: 0-7434-5771-4

First Pocket Books printing May 2003

10   9   8   7   6   5   4   3   2   1

POCKET and colophon are registered trademarks of
Simon & Schuster, Inc.

For information regarding special discounts for bulk purchases,
please contact Simon & Schuster Special Sales at 1-800-456-6798
or business@simonandschuster.com

Printed in the U.S.A.

To my father,
who identified and nurtured all sides of me—
scientific, creative, and humanistic—
and to my mother,
who always believed
that I could do anything

ACKNOWLEDGMENTS

You don't write a book like this one by yourself. In fact, the process of collaborating with and learning from others begins long before you ever glance at your first blank page.

First, I would like to express my appreciation to the attending physicians, midwives, nurses, and residents who shared their knowledge and skills with me during my obstetrics and gynecology residency at University Hospitals' MacDonald House and Cleveland Metropolitan General Hospital in Cleveland, Ohio. Those friends, colleagues, and professors are too numerous to name here, but I sincerely thank them all. Since those days, many others have helped me understand the subtleties of pregnancy and birth. I especially want to thank Patsy Harmon, a certified nurse-midwife; Jill Huppert, M.D.; and certified doulas and childbirth educators Judy Wimmer, R.N., and Karen Kapela. Kudos and thanks also to Dr. John Kennell of Cleveland's Case Western Reserve University School of Medicine, a fine mentor, whose research has demonstrated that humanism really does pay off. And, of course, I am forever grateful to all the families who allowed me to share in some of their most personal experiences. It has been a privilege.

The late Dr. Benjamin Spock is another physician and author I wish to thank. With his ground-breaking book, *Baby and Child Care*, published more than 50 years ago, he gave voice to a philosophy that laid the foundation for a whole new relationship of mutual respect and trust between doctors and families. It was a friend and student of Dr. Spock, pediatrician Laura Jana, who provided me with the advice and encouragement I needed to actually begin writing for expectant mothers and fathers. Dr. Jana was my first editor. She convinced me to join The Dr. Spock Company (where the idea to write this book came to life) and helped fine-tune my understanding of what parents—and parents-to-be—really want to know.

Lisa Rodriguez, R.N., researched and co-wrote many of our original Dr. Spock Company pregnancy articles, which proved to be excellent resources for this book. (They can be found online at *www.drSpock.com*.) Dr. Elisa Ross, a great friend with a gift for clear, simple explanations, served as my valued reviewer. She also kindly allowed me to excerpt portions of the drSpock.com articles we worked on together for certain sections of the book. Melanie McCollum, Ph.D., gave generously of her time and talent to check all the embryology images and descriptions for scientific accuracy. Many thanks also to Dr. Lynn Cates and Dr. Robert Needlman for their insights, and to our team leader, David Markus, and the rest of the content crew at The Dr. Spock Company. My most enthusiastic and sincere thank-you goes to Mona Behan, the best editor (and friend) anyone could possibly wish for, who helped me say just what I wanted to say, only more clearly and with charm.

To my husband and best friend, Dr. Tony Post, I will say only that I am incredibly grateful that you have more confidence in me than I often have in myself. Finally, to our son, Dan Post: a big hug and many thanks for enriching my life, and teaching me how to be a mom.

CONTENTS

INTRODUCTION

Childbirth interested me long before I decided to go into medicine. When I was younger, I read book after book about pregnancy, and was awed and inspired by the birth stories of mothers from different cultures and backgrounds. I wanted to be a midwife, to be present at this intense personal experience. I wanted to go through pregnancy and birth myself.

In my early 20s, I struggled with the decision of whether to become a nurse-midwife or an obstetrician. While I appreciated midwifery's personalized and empowering values and focus on natural childbirth, I realized that being a doctor would allow me more options for caring for my patients. In my medical practice, however, I always have tried not to lose sight of the humanistic, family-focused ideals that originally inspired me. By the time my husband and I had our son, I had delivered thousands of babies. But by going through the incredible experience of giving birth myself, I achieved a depth of understanding of pregnancy and childbirth that nothing else could have provided. Like many other moms and dads, I found pregnancy and parenthood to be a rite of passage that sparked tremendous personal growth, and forever changed my outlook on my family, my work, and myself. My son is now 13, and I still feel as if I'm learning things from him every day that help me be a better person and a better doctor.

In creating this book, I drew upon my more than 15 years' experience as an obstetrician, research on effective medical care for different problems, and advice from other mothers about what made pregnancy more manageable. I've tried to convey this information in a clear, friendly way—the way I talk to patients in my medical practice—and break it into manageable sections to make the march of facts and advice less overwhelming.

HOW TO USE THIS BOOK

Dr. Spock's Pregnancy Guide is divided into chapters that cover each of the nine months of pregnancy, plus a just-in-case 10th chapter on what to expect when pregnancy extends past the due date. The book concludes with a chapter on labor and birth. Each of the chapters is divided into four sections: "About Your Baby," "About You," "Getting Good Care," and "Looking Ahead." Scattered throughout are question-and-answer boxes and a feature called "Parent to Parent," which contains quotes from the lively, honest, and supportive moms and dads who participate in the drSpock.com message boards. Finally, at the end of each chapter you'll find a place to jot down notes about your own pregnancy and questions to ask your doctor or midwife at your next prenatal visit.

Because of the month-by-month organization of the book, topics are placed in a given chapter because you are most likely to experience that particular symptom, problem, or issue during that time period—nausea in Chapter 2, for example, or feeling your baby's first movements in Chapter 5. Some topics, such as travel and weight gain, could have gone anywhere, so I simply chose a chapter that seemed logical. To give you an idea of the wide variety of topics covered and where you might find them, I recommend that you skim through the book from cover to cover, and then go back and read each chapter as you are experiencing that month of pregnancy. Remember to use the index at the back of the book to help you look up anything that doesn't appear where you expect it.

I have tried to focus on the questions my patients most often asked me, and the issues to which I bring a unique perspective. In particular, I have included a lot of information about the choices you make during pregnancy, including how best to achieve the kind of birth experience you want. This is something I feel very strongly about, both as an obstetrician and a woman—an echo, perhaps, of the midwifery ideals that first drew me to this vocation.

My hope is that this book will help diminish the anxiety you may feel about the unknown and unknowable aspects of pregnancy and birth, while providing some useful practical advice. But, above all, I hope these words express some of the awe that I feel about this incredible journey, and help you savor and appreciate your remarkable achievements along the way.

CHAPTER 1

Weeks 0—4

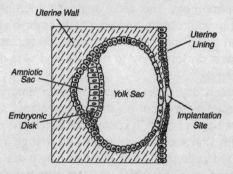

At the end of Week 4 of your pregnancy, the embryo has implanted in the wall of your uterus and consists of two layers of cells, known as the embryonic disk. It's hard to believe that this seemingly simple structure, only about 0.2 millimeters in size, can grow into a baby, but soon the cells will multiply and become specialized, turning into all your child's different body parts.

ABOUT YOUR BABY

The first few weeks of pregnancy can be an exciting time, as you adjust to the idea of being pregnant and start to dream about the new life stirring inside you. In this chapter we'll explore the first month—from the start of your last menstrual cycle to the day that your period would have arrived if you hadn't become pregnant. Most women conceive around Day 14 of their cycles, which means that your embryo will be about two weeks along at the end of this phase (that is, the end of Week 4). In this short time, perhaps before you even notice any changes in your own body, the egg and sperm meet, the cells begin to multiply and implant in your uterus, and your little embryo starts a most amazing journey: the process of becoming a whole new person ready to be born and part of your loving family.

Fourteen days after conception, your embryo is a disk-shaped mass about 0.2 millimeters across, smaller than the head of a pin. It consists of two layers of uniform cells that soon will multiply and change into the specialized cells that form the different parts of the body—that is, some will turn into your baby's eyes, some will start to form his heart, some will become skin cells, and so on. There are hundreds of different cell types, and don't ask how the individual cells know what type they should change into—scientists still do not fully understand how this miraculous process works!

Your body produces everything that your fetus needs

Now and throughout the pregnancy, your baby receives all the nourishment she needs from your body. The food that you eat gets broken down into various nutrients and vitamins, which are transported through your bloodstream. Right now, your embryo is literally bathing in maternal nutrients in your uterus. Later on, when the placenta develops, the nutrients will be carried to the placenta and through the umbilical cord into the fetus's circulation.

COUNTING THE TIME 🐝

Health professionals—as well as most pregnant women—traditionally start to count the weeks of pregnancy from the last menstrual period. This is a holdover from the days when there were no other ways to assess fetal age. When you think about this logically, however, you'll see that it's a bit misleading: When a doctor says that you are four weeks along, the embryo is actually two weeks old, since conception took place around the middle of the month. Confusing, eh? That's why throughout this book we'll stick to the traditional counting system because it's what your doctor or midwife is likely to use.

Take good care, right from the start

In this early stage, there isn't an easy way to check how the embryo is doing in your womb—even ultrasound can't detect it yet. But small as it is, your growing baby still needs you to take very good care of him. You should try to eat well, rest when you are tired, and avoid certain foods and substances that might be harmful. All these things are important throughout your pregnancy, but it's especially crucial during these first weeks, when so many organs are beginning to form. The charts on pages 7–12 will explain the most important things to avoid.

Of course, many moms-to-be don't even know that they are pregnant until they are further along and so couldn't be careful right from the start. If this happened to you, don't panic—most babies still come out just fine! But now that you know that there truly is a baby on board, be sure to do your best to avoid anything that might harm your growing child.

ABOUT YOU

About the only physical change most women notice by the second week after conception may be a little breast tenderness or mild cramping. Occasionally, a woman will have light bleeding (also known as spotting) when the embryo implants in the wall of her uterus, or at the time when she normally would get her period. Some of my patients, however, have sworn to me that they knew the minute they became pregnant because they felt some special emotional or physical change.

A healthy diet includes folate
Eating a healthy diet is one of the most important things you can do to nurture your growing baby—lots of fruits and veggies, and plenty of protein (such as you find in fish, meat, poultry, beans, and soy products). See

Q: Help! I just found out that I'm pregnant and I've been doing a little reading. I have to admit that I'm finding some of the terms in the books and articles confusing. Could you please explain some basic terms, such as uterus, placenta, and amniotic sac? I've heard of these before, but I'm not really sure of the exact definition of each, and what role they play in pregnancy.

A: Sure. I know that all these anatomical terms can be a bit confusing. Simply put, after conception, in which an egg from the mother is joined by a sperm from the father, the fertilized egg burrows into the wall of the **uterus**, a hollow, muscular, stretchable organ in the mother's lower abdomen. Also known as the womb, this is where the fetus will develop throughout the pregnancy. Fluid-filled membranes called the **amniotic sac**, or the bag of waters, surround and cushion the baby inside the uterus. Inside his watery home, the fetus is connected to his mother through his umbilical cord, which extends from his belly button to the **placenta**. The placenta, which resembles a flattened cauliflower, is attached to the inside wall of the uterus, bringing the baby's blood into close contact with his mother's. Through the placenta and the umbilical cord, nutrients and oxygen travel from the mother's body to her baby's, while waste products from the baby are carried back to the mother's body for elimination.

PARENT TO PARENT
"With my last pregnancy and my current one, I 'knew' intuitively before I even missed my first period. The last one, I got dizzy and fell out of bed probably around the time of implantation. This time, I could smell strange odors everywhere."

—**dueinJuly,** AS POSTED ON DRSPOCK.COM

the following chart for some suggestions for a healthy diet. You also should be sure to take folate (also called folic acid), which is a member of the vitamin B family. It has been shown to prevent certain birth defects, including spina bifida, an opening in the back of the spine that can lead to paralysis and other neurological problems. Because folate is so important, even women who eat a good, balanced diet should take 400 micrograms daily; in fact, ideally, you would have started on folate even before becoming pregnant. You can take over-the-counter folate supplements or make sure that your regular multivitamins contain the recommended dosage of this crucial component.

Stay away from certain foods and substances

Just as beneficial substances like nutrients and oxygen flow across the placenta from you to your fetus,

FOODS TO AVOID DURING PREGNANCY			
What to avoid	**Why**	**Alternatives or preventive measures**	**Notes**
Shark, swordfish, tuna steaks, sea bass, and many other large fish	Contain high levels of mercury	Farm-raised trout and catfish, Pacific salmon, and fish sticks are probably safe. Canned tuna once a week also seems to be OK.	Can cause brain or nerve damage when consumed in large amounts. The fetus, which is just developing its nervous system, is likely to be more susceptible than an adult. For more information, check out www.pirg.org/toxics/reports/brainfood.
Raw oysters, clams, and mussels	The illnesses you can get from oysters, clams, and mussels are not specific to pregnancy, but can be severe in anyone, and should be avoided in pregnancy.	Cooking prevents some of these infections, but it cannot prevent the algae-related diseases that are carried on red tides. Avoid *cooked* as well as raw shellfish in warm months, when algae are at their peak.	According to the Food and Drug Administration, undercooked oysters, clams, and mussels are the types of seafood most likely to cause illnesses. These include not only *Salmonella* infection but other types of bacterial, parasitic, and viral infections (including hepatitis A).

Continued

FOODS TO AVOID DURING PREGNANCY

What to avoid	Why	Alternatives or preventive measures	Notes
Raw or under-cooked meat	Toxoplasmosis, a parasitic disease, and a toxic form of the *E. coli* bacterium	When cooking meat, be sure to heat hamburger and pork to an internal temperature of no less than 160°F, and steak to 170° F.	Toxoplasmosis can result in a potentially serious intrauterine fetal infection, leading to premature birth, poor growth, mental retardation, blindness, and other serious problems. *E. coli* contamination can be dangerous for adults and children as well as pregnant women.
Raw chicken	*Salmonella* does not infect the fetus, but the diarrhea and resultant dehydration are not healthy for a pregnant woman.	Cooking chicken well—to a temperature of 180° F—can kill the bacteria.	Utensils used on raw chicken and the plate or board on which you cut it should be put through the dishwasher, where the heat will kill the bacteria. If you don't have a dishwasher, be sure to wash everything with plenty of hot, soapy water.
Raw eggs	*Salmonella*	To eliminate the risk of *Salmonella* infection, always cook your eggs well before eating, and ask if raw eggs are used in any dish when you are dining out.	Risky foods include Caesar salad (if it's made with raw eggs; many versions aren't) and eggnog. It is also a good idea to resist the temptation to taste batter containing raw eggs before cooking.

Continued

FOODS TO AVOID DURING PREGNANCY

What to avoid	Why	Alternatives or preventive measures	Notes
Unpasteurized milk and soft unpasteurized cheeses (such as Brie, Camembert, and Mexican-style cheeses like *queso fresco*)	*Listeria*	Most cheeses available in the United States are pasteurized, but be sure to check the label.	While adults with listeriosis often show no signs of infection or simply develop flulike symptoms, *Listeria* bacteria have the ability to cross the placenta and infect the fetus. Listeriosis has been known to cause miscarriage, premature birth, and serious infections.
Pâté	*Listeria*	Don't eat pâté until after you have the baby.	See above.
Unwashed vegetables	Toxoplasmosis, *Listeria, E. coli, Salmonella*	Wash all veggies.	See above. Vegetables that are not washed have the potential to transmit these organisms, since they can contaminate the soil in which the vegetables were grown. For the same reason, pregnant women should wear gloves when gardening, and should wash their hands afterward.

Continued

SUBSTANCES TO AVOID DURING PREGNANCY

What to avoid	Why	Alternatives or preventive measures	Notes
Medications	While many medications are probably safe, most haven't been tested for use in pregnancy (see Chapter 3).	If you are sick or in pain, try nonmedical treatments first. Before taking any medication, you should check with your doctor.	The most vulnerable time for the fetus is during the first trimester.
Alcoholic beverages	Alcohol has been shown to cause birth defects after low-level repeated use (as little as three drinks a day) or occasional binge drinking. This is true throughout pregnancy, but it is particularly damaging in the first trimester. Worldwide, alcohol is probably the greatest single cause of birth defects.	It's probably best not to drink, even a little—after all, what other proven fetal toxin would you let pass your lips during pregnancy? If you drink regularly, or have trouble quitting on your own, get help before becoming pregnant or as soon as you know you are expecting.	The main features of fetal alcohol syndrome (FAS) are poor growth, abnormal facial features, and cognitive problems ranging from trouble with learning and attention to more severe mental retardation. Many children who don't seem to have the full FAS picture may have a milder form, with learning problems but not the physical signs.
Cigarettes	The ill effects are due to nicotine (which causes spasm of the arteries that provide oxygen	Quit! (See box on page 16.) But while any smoking is bad, going through less than half a pack a day is definitely	The emotional repercussions of smoking during pregnancy can be severe: Mothers who have smoking-related complications

Continued

SUBSTANCES TO AVOID DURING PREGNANCY

What to avoid	Why	Alternatives or preventive measures	Notes
Cigarettes	and nutrients to the baby), carbon monoxide (which also interferes with oxygen delivery), and other toxins. Miscarriage, placental abruption, premature rupture of the membranes, premature birth, and low birth weight all have been shown to be more prevalent in the pregnancies of smokers.	better than a heavier habit. The best outcomes for babies occur when the mothers don't smoke at all or quit in the first trimester.	have to deal with the bad outcomes plus guilt over having contributed to the suffering of their families. Exposure to second-hand smoke in the home poses a real risk as well. And on top of all that, if a parent smokes, a child is more likely to become a smoker.
Cocaine	Cocaine use can result in prematurity, low birth weight, and a dangerous birth complication in which the placenta separates from the uterus prematurely. In rare cases, cocaine may damage internal fetal organs.	Quit, and if you have trouble quitting on your own, get help.	Across the board, researchers have found that, as a group, children exposed to cocaine in the womb have lower IQ scores and more learning, emotional, and behavior problems than children born to mothers who didn't use the drug.

Continued

SUBSTANCES TO AVOID DURING PREGNANCY			
What to avoid	Why	Alternatives or preventive measures	Notes
Marijuana	Marijuana may interfere with fetal growth and cause subtle problems in brain development.	The wise thing to do is to avoid recreational drugs altogether.	

so too can harmful chemicals, parasites, viruses, and bacteria. Even certain foods that are usually safe to eat can prove harmful to a fetus. The preceding charts list the most common foods and substances to avoid, and explain the dangers they pose to your growing child. The list may seem long and a little daunting, but keep in mind that there are still plenty of other delicious foods that will do you and your baby a world of good.

The verdict's still out on some foods
Many doctors and scientists now believe that some of the foods and ingredients that were once considered unsafe during pregnancy actually may not be so bad after all:

- **Aspartame.** Aspartame, an artificial sweetener found in NutraSweet and many other products, contains phenylalanine, an amino acid (amino acids are the building blocks of protein) that is toxic for children with the rare genetic condition phenylketonuria (PKU). Even if your baby has PKU, your body would break down any phenylalanine you eat before it crossed the placenta, rendering it harmless to your fetus. However, the most prudent advice is to consume aspartame only in moderation (which is a good idea even if you're not pregnant).

- **Caffeine.** In addition to coffee and some teas, many soft drinks and chocolate products contain caffeine, and large amounts of this substance have been linked to miscarriages in the first trimester. However, *one* caffeinated drink a day has never been shown to be damaging, so if you crave a daily cup of coffee or an occasional cola drink, it's probably just fine.

- **Sushi.** This Japanese delicacy has become very popular in the United States; in fact, if they like the type of sushi made with raw fish, many of my patients find it one of the hardest things to give up when they become pregnant! If such sushi isn't handled properly or is contaminated with bacteria, viruses, or parasites, yes, it can be quite dangerous indeed, and not just to pregnant women. But there have been few reports of illness resulting from sushi served in restaurants staffed by trained sushi chefs, who know how to buy, store, and serve the fish and spot signs of contamination. It may be prudent not to prepare sushi at home, however, unless you can be certain of the freshness of the fish and know how to check it for parasites or other problems. Besides, you can always enjoy the types of sushi made with cooked fish or vegetables.

Let your spouse change the kitty litter for a while

In addition to staying away from certain foods and substances like cigarettes and alcohol, there are a few other things you should avoid while you're pregnant:

- **X rays.** High amounts of radiation can cause miscarriage or birth defects. If you're pregnant—or are trying to become pregnant—be sure to speak up before getting x-rayed, even routine dental X rays. X rays involving the lower part of your body are especially important to avoid if you can. Sometimes there are medical reasons why you might need to have an X ray despite your pregnancy, but you should *always* tell the doctor or technician about your condition.

- **Fever or getting overheated.** If your body temperature climbs too high, it may increase the risk of birth defects in your baby. If you develop a fever, particularly in your first trimester, you can take acetaminophen (such as found in Tylenol) to bring it down (see page 64). On hot days, try to stay cool and drink lots of water. And stay out of any hot tub that's heated to more than 101 degrees: Although some research has shown that pregnant women instinctively tend to get out of the tub as soon as their body temperatures rise, it's better not to take any chances.

- **The litter box.** Cat feces can harbor the protozoan that causes toxoplasmosis, a disease that doesn't bother adults very much but can have devastating effects on a fetus, including brain damage and blindness. This is especially true if the fetus is infected early in the pregnancy. If you have a cat, be sure to wash your hands after petting your animal, and get someone else to change the kitty litter. Some people, though, have developed immunity to this common disease, which also would protect their fetuses; your doctor can do a blood test to find out if this is true in your case.

- **Rubella, chickenpox, cytomegalovirus (CMV), fifth disease (slapped cheek disease).** These diseases can pose a variety of serious risks to fetuses. If you had chickenpox or were vaccinated, you—and your fetus—are probably protected from infection. You also may have developed immunity to rubella (also known as German measles); your practitioner will test you. If you work with children in a school, daycare center, or medical setting, consider asking your practitioner to do a blood test to see if you are immune to CMV and parvovirus (which causes fifth disease). And just as with many other infectious diseases, your best defense is to wash your hands frequently with soap and water.

KICKING THE CIGARETTE HABIT 🚴

To nonsmokers, it's obvious that pregnant women shouldn't smoke. But for smokers, the prospect of quitting can be so dreadful that many try to ignore the danger that their habit poses for their babies. The danger is quite real, however, and if you smoke, you really should try to quit, preferably in the first trimester. I'm not trying to lecture you, but in my practice I've seen firsthand the damage that a pregnant woman's smoking can inflict on her fetus, and it breaks my heart.

Sometimes it takes several attempts before a person finally kicks the habit for good, so don't feel discouraged if you've tried before and failed. Often I find that getting pregnant gives my patients who were smokers the extra motivation they need.

In pregnancy, you can stop smoking cold turkey or you can slowly decrease the number of cigarettes you have each day over a few weeks. You also can take bupropion (Zyban), a prescription medication that helps take the edge off cravings. Although nicotine replacement therapy (such as the patch or gum) is controversial (after all, you're still introducing some nicotine into the baby's system), it's safer than smoking, and the goal would be to get off the replacement within a few weeks, too.

For specific ideas on how to quit, talk to your healthcare practitioner. You also might want to check out the excellent articles on the National Cancer Institute website at http://rex.nci.nih.gov/ NCI_Pub_Interface/Clearing_the_Air/clearing.html

GETTING GOOD CARE

In an ideal world, your first "prenatal" visit would have occurred at least three months *before* you became pregnant (known as a pre-conception visit). That's because a baby's organs start to form within 17 days after conception, and a lot will have happened by the time of a typical first prenatal appointment, which usually takes place when you already are 6 to 10 weeks along.

A pre-conception visit often is useful for recognizing factors that can affect the timing of a pregnancy, or even the decision whether or not to become pregnant at all. This is particularly true for women with significant health problems (such as diabetes, epilepsy, and congenital heart disease) and for couples with genetic risk factors. There are routine tests available to see if you carry certain genetic diseases. While these can be done in early pregnancy, you may feel better able to deal with the results if the tests are performed before you become pregnant.

Maternity practitioners range from doctors to lay midwives

Once you learn that you're pregnant, you may find yourself daydreaming about baby names and nursery decor, but do remember that you have some pressing tasks at hand, including the selection of a maternity-care practitioner if you don't already have one. There are many factors to consider—everything from the type of insurance the practice accepts to the type of birth setting you want. To help you understand your options, here's some information on the types of practitioners who provide maternity care, as well as the different types of group practices and birth settings:

- **Obstetrician**. Obstetricians, or OBs for short, have completed four years of medical school followed by at least four years of training in normal and high-risk obstetrics, as well as other aspects of women's health. They must be licensed physicians and may be board certified in obstetrics and gynecology. (*Board certified* means that a doctor passed specialized exams after completing residency.) OBs can perform the full range of deliveries: regular vaginal births, operative vaginal deliveries (vacuum and/or forceps), and cesareans. They usually deliver in hospitals. Obstetricians vary widely in their childbirth philosophies: Some are very medically oriented, while others are exceptionally supportive of keeping things as natural as possible. To get more information, contact the American College of Obstetricians and Gynecologists at *www.ACOG.org*.

- **Family physician.** Family doctors have had four years of medical school and usually have had three years of residency training in family care, including pediatrics, adult internal medicine, and obstetrics. All family physicians (FPs) must be licensed doctors and may be board certified. These doctors can do regular vaginal deliveries, and with further training, some can do operative vaginal deliveries. In some parts of the country, they also perform cesareans. Most FPs collaborate with an obstetrician if the pregnancy or the labor becomes complicated. FPs also can take care of your baby after birth, and can provide regular medical care for you and your family. To get more information, contact the American Academy of Family Physicians at *www.familydoctor.org*.

- **Certified nurse-midwife (CNM).** A certified nurse-midwife is a registered nurse with at least two or three years' additional training in normal obstetrics and women's health care; many also have a master's degree in nursing. Every CNM must be licensed as a nurse and must pass other exams to be certified as a nurse-midwife. Their extensive training for the care of healthy, low-risk women gives nurse-midwives a unique perspective on the normal experiences of pregnancy, labor, and birth. Most nurse-midwives are oriented toward natural childbirth and will stay with you through your labor, similar to a doula (see page 179). Certified nurse-midwives can deliver babies in hospitals or birth centers, and some attend home births. They practice in collaboration with a physician, in case complications develop. To get more information, contact the American College of Nurse-Midwives at *www.acnm.org*.

- **Certified midwife.** A certified midwife is a new category of practitioner with training similar to that of nurse-midwives. Certified midwives must pass the same exams as certified nurse-midwives, but they weren't trained as nurses. Currently, this certification is recognized only in some states. To get more information, contact the American College of Nurse-Midwives at *www.acnm.org*.

- **Lay midwife.** Not every midwife is certified. Lay midwives learn their pregnancy-care and childbirth skills as apprentices to other, more experienced lay midwives; they are not certified or regulated by the government in most states. This means that there is no requirement concerning specific training or tests to assess their competence. Lay midwives normally attend only home births, and don't have credentials to attend births in birth centers or hospitals. A lay midwife should have backup from a physician, in case complications develop. To get more information, contact the Midwives Alliance of North America at *www.mana.org*.

- **Perinatologist.** A perinatologist, or maternal-fetal medicine specialist, is an OB who has done an extra fellowship for two or three years *after* becoming an obstetrician. These specialists focus on medically complicated, high-risk pregnancies. Perinatologists always practice in hospitals, often in teaching hospitals that are set up to take care of difficult pregnancies and severely ill babies. To get more information, contact the Society for Maternal Fetal Medicine at *www.smfm.org*.

WATER BIRTHS 🌿

In a water birth, a woman spends much of her labor and gives birth in a big tub of warm water, which seems to provide many laboring women with a tremendous sense of relaxation and pain relief. Water births are for women who want natural, unmedicated childbirth—no epidurals (see page 154) in the tub!

If such a birth option appeals to you, you should plan well ahead. You'll need to find a maternity-care practitioner who is experienced in water births, and the facility in which you will deliver should be equipped to monitor the progress and condition of you and your baby in the tub. If a hospital or birth center doesn't provide tubs, you may be able to rent one for your delivery. You should note that there hasn't been a lot of safety research comparing water births to the usual type of deliveries, making some practitioners leery of them. You also should be aware that many practitioners are open to the idea of women laboring in a bathtub, but believe that it is safer to perform the actual delivery out of the water.

Childbirth settings provide different experiences

- **Hospitals.** In the United States, most babies are born in hospitals. Obstetricians, family practitioners, and nurse-midwives all can deliver babies in the hospital. There are different types: Teaching hospitals generally have the greatest availability of specialists and high-tech medical treatments, but they often have more people, including trainees like residents and students, involved in your care. Community hospitals generally don't have many students and residents, but they often have higher cesarean rates than teaching hospitals. Individual hospitals differ in their epidural and cesarean rates and the availability of anesthesia and emergency consultation. Hospitals differ, too, in the level of care that the nursery can provide to newborns without having to transfer them to another location, in their general protocols and rules, and in their response to individualized birth plans.

In addition to traditional hospital rooms, many hospitals now have low-tech labor/delivery/recovery rooms for uncomplicated births. Some even try to create a homelike setting with such amenities as rocking chairs, pretty quilts and drapes, and soothing murals. Many hospitals offer tours for expectant parents. Ask your practitioner about the settings in which she delivers, and take a look at the ones that appeal to you.

• **Birth centers.** Birth centers may be freestanding or physically attached to a hospital. They offer a more homelike environment than hospitals, and usually provide only natural, unmedicated childbirth. If a complication arises (such as the need for a cesarean), the woman or the newborn may be transferred to a hospital; in fact, about 10 percent of birth-center moms end up being transferred to a hospital before their babies are born.

- **Home.** Home birth is not a common choice in the United States today. Most obstetricians (and most American parents) believe that childbirth at home is not safe. Couples who choose home birth generally want to take active responsibility for their own health-care and may feel safer at home than in the hospital. Many home births are attended by lay midwives, since nurse-midwives often find it difficult to get malpractice insurance if they participate in home births. If you are considering a home birth, be sure to educate yourself about the risks, as well as potential benefits, of giving birth in such a low-tech, isolated setting.

Group practices are the norm

Most practitioners do not work 24/7—hey, even doctors sometimes have personal lives. It's likely that your practitioner is part of a group practice and that someone else may be on call when your baby decides to arrive. When choosing a practice, therefore, consider asking questions such as:

- Does the practice accept my medical insurance?
- At which hospitals do the practitioners have admitting privileges (i.e., where will I be able to deliver my baby)?
- Will I see all members of the group on a rotating basis during my prenatal care?
- If I see primarily one practitioner, who else in the practice might deliver the baby? Will I meet him during my prenatal visits?

- What are the chances that my primary practitioner will be there for me in labor?
- Do the other practitioners have a similar philosophy and personal style?
- (And if you go to a family doctor or nurse-midwife) What are the arrangements if I need an obstetrician due to a complication in the pregnancy or birth?

There aren't "right" answers to these questions. Just be sure that you are comfortable with the answers provided to you.

LOOKING AHEAD

Although you may have just found out that you're pregnant, no doubt your mind is racing ahead to the Big Day, the moment when your child makes his debut into the world. If you're like many moms-to-be, you might become keenly interested in knowing (maybe even obsessed by) your due date. Aside from helping you plan, identifying the due date is important because some key prenatal tests need to be performed at specific times during your pregnancy.

Due dates can be tricky to calculate
The most accurate method to calculate your due date is to find the date 266 days after you conceived. But you may not know exactly when that little sperm hooked up with that little egg, and then things get trickier.

Women with average menstrual cycles tend to get

their period every 28 days, so conception is likely to have occurred on Day 14. In women with short cycles (22 to 24 days), ovulation can occur as early as Day 8 or 9. Women with longer cycles (up to 35 days) might ovulate as late as Day 21 or so. But whether your cycle is short, long, or average, it is always 14 days *from* ovulation to the *next* menstrual cycle. So if your cycle is regular (that is, always the same length), you can subtract 14 days from when your period was due to determine the most likely date of conception. (Women with irregular cycles are out of luck with this method, since the time you ovulate varies from month to month.)

Another way to estimate your due date is to start with the first day of your last menstrual cycle. Subtract three months and add seven days. For example, if your last period began on June 7, your due date would be March 14. This method is most accurate if you're sure about the date of your last period and your cycles are approximately 28 days long.

I know that this can be confusing, but your doctor or midwife will help you calculate your due date. And if you're not sure of the day your last period began, your practitioner probably will do an ultrasound at some point to help estimate how far along you might be.

Babies don't respect due dates

Now that you've done all the math to figure out your due date, I hesitate to tell you that your baby probably will decide to arrive earlier or later. Only 5 percent of all babies are born on their official due dates—5 percent! Eighty percent arrive within two weeks before or after their due dates, so you have a good month's window to consider.

A couple often finds it very difficult if the due date passes and their baby still shows no signs of showing up. It's even more stressful when friends and relatives, with the best of intentions, start asking why the baby hasn't yet arrived. Since nearly half of all babies are born after their due dates, it pays to be a little vague when announcing yours. For example, when someone asks when the baby is due, instead of saying, "July 23," you might say, "The end of July."

Think about genetic testing

As you prepare for your first prenatal appointment, be aware that your practitioner is likely to talk with you about genetic testing. Some types of genetic tests can be done on the parents, while others must involve the fetus and can't be done until the third to fifth month of pregnancy. We'll cover the second type in Chapter 4, but it's good to understand a little about parental genetic testing before you walk in for your first prenatal visit.

In case you've forgotten the genetics you learned in school, let me refresh your memory about the basics: All humans have two genes for nearly every character-istic we possess, inheriting one from our mother and one from our father. With some diseases, all it takes is for one of the genes to be faulty to produce the illness; other types of diseases require that both genes carry the trait. This means you can't assume that since you and your partner don't have a particular medical condi-tion, your baby won't; genetic testing often is the only way to tell if a person carries the gene for a particular illness.

Parental genetic testing is usually done either during a pre-conception visit or very early in pregnancy, and it's become very common. For example, the American College of Obstetricians and Gynecologists now recommends that most newly pregnant couples (or those planning a pregnancy) be offered testing for the gene that causes cystic fibrosis, a serious disease that occurs in 1 in 2,500 children in the United States. Couples also may be screened for other genetic problems such as Tay-Sachs disease, a devastating neurological condition, and sickle cell disease, a severe form of anemia with far-reaching medical consequences.

If your family history or ethnic or racial makeup puts you in a high-risk group for certain conditions, your practitioner may urge you to be tested. Some couples welcome the chance to check for potential problems, while others decline the screening, perhaps because they intend to have the baby no matter what the tests might reveal. Remember that it's *your* choice, and talking with your partner about the possibilities and options ahead of time will help you be prepared when your practitioner brings up the subject.

NOTES

Use this space to jot down observations about your
pregnancy or questions to ask your healthcare practitioner at your next visit:

_____

_____

_____

_____

_____

_____

_____

_____

_____

_____

_____

_____

CHAPTER 2

Weeks 5—8

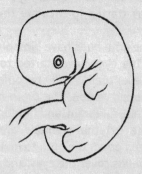

Around Week 7, the embryo has a head and a tail. The latter will quickly disappear, as some of the cells turn into other body parts while others are simply reabsorbed. The little being also has sprouted small buds that will grow into limbs, and the tiny heart is already beating. The embryo is about 10 millimeters long—a bit less than ½ inch.

ABOUT YOUR BABY

Around Week 5—probably the time that you missed your first period—your embryo develops a third cell layer; each of these outer, middle, and inner layers is destined to become a different part of your baby's body. Cells continue to organize, and the neural tube,

which will evolve into the brain and spinal cord, is starting to form.

At Week 6, your embryo is about ¼ inch long. The
heart, which started to beat just 22 days after conception, is too small to hear, even with amplification, but it
can sometimes be seen as a flickering on an ultrasound
screen. Blood has started to circulate through the tiny
body.

By Week 7, the limb buds have blossomed into teeny
arms and legs. The eyes have started to form, and an
opening that eventually will become the mouth
appears in the head region. The brain now has three
divisions (forebrain, midbrain, and hindbrain), as it does
in an adult. The external genitals are forming but
haven't yet started down the path to male or female.

In Week 8, eyelids cover the eyes, and the lens starts
to develop. The beginning of a nose appears, and fingers and toes begin to form. Your embryo's brain is
growing rapidly, causing a noticeable bulge. The
embryo is not quite one inch in length—not very big, I
know, but rather impressive, considering it's tripled its
size in about two weeks.

ABOUT YOU

You are now in the thick of the first trimester, the first
third of pregnancy. By this time you're probably well
acquainted with some of the symptoms of early pregnancy, such as nausea and fatigue. But take heart:
These common nuisances usually peak around Week 9
and then start to fade away.

You're likely to have noticed emotional symptoms as well. Even women with planned and desired pregnancies can have mixed feelings at this point, as they see their relationships, their lives, and their bodies start to change. Your emotions may swing between excitement and worry, euphoria and the blues (as might your partner's—see page 49). The whole thing may seem unreal. But no matter how you feel, your little embryo is developing at an amazing rate, with new organs forming every week.

Just like your embryo, your body is undergoing a wondrous transformation. Most women have symptoms that tell them something big is happening—some welcome, others not so pleasant. Here are some of the physical and emotional changes you may notice in this month:

- breast tenderness, an increase in breast size, and a darkening of the area surrounding the nipple called the areola (pronounced air-ee-OH-la)
- a cessation of your menstrual periods (although some women experience a little spotting in the first month or so)
- cramps, similar to menstrual cramps: This is normal in early pregnancy, but if the cramping is severe or accompanied by vaginal bleeding, contact your practitioner.
- unusual fatigue: You often may need to take a nap in the afternoon or go to bed in the early evening.
- frequent urination

- an unusual sensitivity to certain odors
- nausea and vomiting: If your so-called morning sickness is excessive, you may even lose some weight.
- an increase in appetite or a craving for certain foods
- weight gain: Although your embryo is still very small, your blood volume increases and your fat stores go up, in preparation for carrying the baby.
- constipation
- heartburn
- dizziness or feelings of faintness
- emotional instability, such as mood swings and irritability, or difficulty concentrating.

Some mothers-to-be feel very different during early pregnancy, while others hardly notice any changes. You may react one way in your first pregnancy, and just the opposite the second time around. Many symptoms and conditions will disappear as the months pass, while others may continue until you deliver your baby. If your symptoms are making you miserable, there are some things you can do to relieve them, but also try to remind yourself that these are signs of your own personal miracle in the making.

Fatigue affects most moms-to-be in the first trimester

Early in pregnancy, most women feel immensely tired. Many find that they can't get through the day without a nap, or that they go to sleep as soon as they get home from work. Why is this so? No one knows for sure, but there is probably a reason we humans have developed this tendency since it is so universal. Perhaps it is a signal for us to start listening to our bodies and treating ourselves well early in pregnancy. After all, we are hard at work creating a whole new being.

To feel more rested and energetic:

- Try to get some exercise to boost your energy level, even though it can be difficult to get started. At least, try to take a walk every day.

- Go to bed earlier and get up a little later if possible.

- Eat healthful, nutritious meals (including breakfast as often as you can).

- Get help at home with cleaning, cooking, or tending the kids.

- At work, try to take short breaks and find a quiet place where you can put up your feet and close your eyes for a few minutes. Rest during your lunch break, but make sure that you leave enough time to eat.

- If you have other children, you may find that you are even more fatigued this time around, and it can be hard to get a break to rest. Try to lie down at the same time your other children are napping. If they don't nap, tell them it's quiet time and Mommy needs to rest.

Do the best you can to get through this difficult time. The good news is that most women find that they have much more energy by Month 4, the start of their second trimester.

PARENT TO PARENT

"Three days before I took my home pregnancy test, I was eating and discovered that I had lost my taste for a dish I always had loved. I knew that something was wrong. Still, to this day, I get nauseous every time I smell fettuccine Alfredo."

—**branvick,** AS POSTED ON DRSPOCK.COM

Food and the first trimester

Many women experience a love-hate relationship with food in the first trimester. You may feel ravenous all the time, or perhaps even the faintest whiff of a tuna-fish sandwich makes your stomach flip-flop. Maybe you're craving things you never had a taste for previously, or find yourself eating the same familiar comfort foods over and over. You know that you need to eat well for the baby's sake, but morning sickness can make a healthy diet seem like an impossible goal.

Nausea can be a fact of life in early pregnancy

What many people often call morning sickness is often better named "evening sickness" or even "every-minute-of-the-day sickness." While the lucky few sail through pregnancy without a single queasy moment, 50 to 90 percent of all pregnant women experience some degree of nausea and vomiting. Fortunately, for most, nausea is a first-trimester problem, peaking at Week 9 or 10 and completely gone by Week 14 or so. I know that this is small consolation when you're feeling miserable, but I promise that most moms-to-be feel much better by the middle of their pregnancies.

Many women worry that the very act of vomiting may hurt their babies, but fetuses are well protected in the uterus, so this type of physical strain isn't going to cause them any harm. However, if you get dehydrated or go into a starvation state, it can be very unhealthy. Some women need brief hospital treatment for intravenous fluids and antinausea medications if their condition becomes serious. This severe form of nausea and vomiting is called *hyperemesis gravidarum*.

To deal with nausea and vomiting:

- **Eat when you are able and see what works for you.** Try eating bland dry foods, and avoid fatty or spicy foods. It is OK to eat a less than perfectly balanced diet in the first trimester. Consume your liquids

separately from dry foods. Try sports drinks, water,
clear juices, Kool-Aid, or noncaffeinated tea. Avoid
carbonated beverages that fill up your stomach. Try
eating lots of little meals. If you tend to feel sick
when you first wake up, leave crackers or dry cereal
next to the bed for a quick, stomach-settling snack
before rising. Keep healthy snacks with you all day
to nibble on when you feel queasy or to ward off
nausea in the first place. If you are unable to keep
anything down, or if you notice signs of dehydration, such as lightheadedness, severe thirst, or
infrequent urination, call your healthcare practitioner.

- **Remember that prenatal vitamins sometimes
  worsen nausea.** While folic acid is necessary, especially early in pregnancy, many women find a small,
  stand-alone folate supplement easier to tolerate
  than a multivitamin pill. If your vitamins seem to be
  contributing to your nausea, ask your practitioner if
  it is all right to temporarily replace prenatal vitamins with just folate pills.

- **Try some sensible alternative treatments.** Your
  healthcare practitioner may be able to suggest
  some natural measures to treat nausea that are not
  known to pose any risks for the fetus. For example,
  some women swear by acupressure or acupuncture
  treatments by trained professionals, and wrist-
  bands that stimulate acupressure points (often
  marketed for seasickness) are available at most
  drugstores or travel stores. Ginger root is used for
  nausea in many traditional cultures, and some

women take fresh grated ginger or ginger tablets. The pill form may contain other ingredients or contaminants, so fresh ginger is probably a safer choice. Try brewing tea from grated ginger or adding it to recipes.

- **If your nausea is severe, talk to your doctor about medications.** Right now, Emetrol is the only nausea medication approved for use in pregnancy in the United States. It is available over the counter and is soothing to the stomach. A prescription medication called Bendectin was available in the 1970s and 80s and was shown to be safe in pregnancy, but the company stopped marketing it in the United States due to apparently unwarranted lawsuits. (A similar product is still sold in Canada under the name of Diclectin.) However, your doctor may be able to suggest a way to duplicate the active ingredients in this product using vitamins and over-the-counter medications. Talk to your practitioner and see if she thinks this might be safe for you.

Prescription medications like prochlorperazine (Compazine) and promethazine (Phenergan) can be used if the benefits outweigh possible risks, but these have not been clearly shown to be safe in pregnancy. Acid-blocking medications such as famotidine (Pepcid), cimetidine (Tagamet), and ranitidine (Zantac) are sometimes helpful and are probably safe. Metoclopramide (Reglan) causes your stomach to empty quickly after eating and alleviates nausea; it, too, seems to be safe in pregnancy. Ondansetron (Zofran), an expensive but very effective medicine often used to treat nausea resulting from chemotherapy, also can be used in certain situations.

A good diet is important—but all in good time

If you find it difficult even coming close to eating a balanced diet in your first trimester, rest assured that you are not alone. To ward off queasiness, some women snack all the time (and not necessarily on the healthiest stuff) and quickly put on a lot of pounds. Others are hardly able to get anything down and actually lose weight. And for many mothers-to-be, only a limited number of foods seem tolerable.

But don't worry. Getting enough folate (see page 4) and preventing malnutrition and dehydration are the most important considerations in the first trimester. If a perfectly balanced diet were that important, we wouldn't have evolved to feel so nauseated during pregnancy!

Many mothers-to-be wonder whether or not they are making the best nutritional choices for their developing babies. The good news is that most fetuses can make do with what they're given and grow well despite a mom's less-than-stellar diet. That said, it's still wise to take in enough good nutrition for both of you. As soon as the nausea has diminished and you feel ready to eat more healthfully, drink lots of fluids and try to follow the USDA food pyramid guidelines: That is, eat plenty of whole grains, fruits, and veggies; a moderate amount of dairy and meat (or other sources of protein); and sparing amounts of fats and sweets.

THE CAUSES OF NAUSEA AND VOMITING 🐝

We can't explain why some pregnant women feel fine and others are green for months. Even the same woman may feel vastly different in each pregnancy. However, there does seem to be some relationship between nausea and the level of the pregnancy hormone human chorionic gonadotropin, a mouthful usually just referred to as hCG. In twin pregnancies and in other situations in which the hCG is greater than usual, nausea and vomiting tend to be worse.

Many women experience vaginal bleeding in early pregnancy

First-trimester bleeding occurs in about one in four pregnancies. It may vary from a small amount of spotting to heavy bleeding with clots and cramps. Occasionally the bleeding comes and goes, and you may think that you're still getting your periods.

Many mothers-to-be get a few days of bleeding right around the time that the embryo is burrowing into the wall of the uterus. On average, this occurs five days after conception and may be confused with a menstrual period, especially if you're not keeping close track of your cycles. This implantation bleeding is normal and is not a sign of any problem with the pregnancy. The biggest problem with implantation bleeding is that it can lead to a mistakenly later due date if it is counted as a menstrual period. The real last period from which the due date should be calculated would be the prior one.

Technically, any bleeding in the first half of pregnancy is defined as a threatened miscarriage or (in medical terms) threatened abortion. But don't let these terms alarm you: More than half the women who have some bleeding in early pregnancy go on to have a healthy baby.

If you are having mild first-trimester bleeding, you should let your practitioner know, but there's no need to panic. It is more urgent to call your practitioner if you have bleeding heavier than your normal period, severe cramps, lower abdominal pain, or fever. These can be signs of miscarriage or another pregnancy complication such as an ectopic pregnancy, in which the fertilized egg starts developing outside the uterus (see page 41). Call your doctor night or day if these symptoms arise. She may give you a physical exam and usually will order an ultrasound or a blood test to see if the pregnancy is OK. When there is bleeding, germs can get up into the uterus more easily, so it is best to put nothing into your vagina until the bleeding has stopped; that means no douching, no tampons, and no intercourse. You will be able to resume sexual relations when your bleeding has resolved. Although this surprises many women, bed rest is generally not necessary.

Miscarriage in the first trimester

Miscarriage (technically called spontaneous abortion) is defined as the loss of a pregnancy before 20 weeks' gestation. About one in eight pregnancies ends in miscar-

---

THE HEARTBREAK OF ECTOPIC PREGNANCY

In about 1 out of 100 pregnancies, instead of making its way to the uterus, the fertilized egg implants itself in one of the two fallopian tubes, which connect the ovaries to the uterus. This situation is known as an ectopic, or tubal, pregnancy. The fallopian tubes cannot stretch like the uterus to accommodate a growing embryo, nor can they provide the necessary nutrients. When an egg mistakenly implants itself in one of these tubes, it typically results in a miscarriage, and in some cases, a tear in the tube (called a ruptured ectopic). Ectopic pregnancies often cause abdominal pain and occasionally lead to internal bleeding. They are more frequent in women who have had prior ectopic pregnancies or who have sustained damage to their fallopian tubes. Most of the time, a tubal pregnancy can be diagnosed and treated with medicine or surgery before the situation poses a serious threat to the mother's health. Unfortunately, an ectopic pregnancy is not viable, and the fetus cannot be transplanted and saved.

---

riage. The rate is even higher for older mothers or fathers. Actually, this number is an underestimate, since some women miscarry before they know they are pregnant, and interpret the miscarriage bleeding as a menstrual period. The majority of miscarriages occur before

12 weeks. After 12 weeks, if a good heartbeat is heard or the pregnancy looks normal on ultrasound, the chance of miscarriage goes down to about 1 percent.

Some miscarriages occur all at once, with heavy bleeding and cramping, passing tissue from the vagina, and then resolution of the symptoms over 6 to 12 hours. In this case, a woman should see her practitioner within a day or two for an examination to be sure that nothing needs to be done medically. Although I know this can be hard to do, it is helpful if she collects any tissue (red, gray, or white solid material) that is passed and keeps it in a clean jar in the refrigerator to show the doctor. The woman's blood type will be checked, and if she is Rh-negative, she may be given an injection of RhoGam in case her blood and the embryo's are incompatible; it helps prevent the mother from developing antibodies that could harm a future pregnancy (see page 149–152).

Sometimes physical examination, ultrasound, or results of blood hormone levels indicate that a miscarriage is still in progress. In these cases, some of the placental tissue may still remain inside the uterus and may require removal with a small vacuum tube, a surgical procedure called dilation and curettage (D & C). This is usually done in an outpatient surgery center or in a hospital under light anesthesia.

Parents-to-be often are devastated if they lose a pregnancy. Many women end up blaming themselves for something they did or did not do—"I should have stayed in bed," they worry, or "I wasn't eating right." But the truth is that, in most cases, whether or not a woman is going to miscarry is out of her hands, and there was nothing she could have done to prevent it. Many miscarriages are caused by chromosomal problems or by abnormal fetal development; it's very sad for the parents, but it's nature's way of avoiding the birth of some severely damaged babies.

If you have endured a miscarriage, you may find it hard to believe, but your chances for a healthy pregnancy the next time around are excellent if it was your first miscarriage and it occurred in the first trimester. Once you become pregnant again, in most cases you are no more at risk of miscarriage than anyone else. If you have had two consecutive losses, or three or more total losses interspersed with normal pregnancies, discuss with your practitioner whether a workup for causes of recurrent miscarriage might be helpful.

The emotional toll of a threatened or actual miscarriage

Finding out that a pregnancy may not be progressing as you had anticipated can lead to feelings of anxiety, hopelessness, fear, sadness, desperation, or anger—or any combination of these emotions. While ultrasound is helpful in determining the state of your pregnancy, it also can put you face-to-face with bad news in an unfamiliar medical office without your family members or regular practitioner to comfort you. Sometimes the ultrasound staff can't give you information on the spot because they don't know your medical situation or what the next step would be in your care. In this case, they may refer you back to your doctor, which can feel like a cruel delay when you are worrying. While doubts and fears may be causing you great pain, keep in mind that the destiny of this pregnancy is already determined. You need answers for your peace of mind or so your grieving can begin, but there is nothing at this point that you can do to change fate. When you get home, gather those around you who can give you sustenance and support in the coming days.

GETTING GOOD CARE

Getting good prenatal medical care is a chance to start being a concerned parent even before your baby is born. There are substantial health benefits: Research has shown that women who see a doctor or nurse-midwife for regular prenatal checkups are less likely to have premature and low-birth-weight babies than those who do not. Many women look forward to their appointments, knowing that it's a chance to ask questions of their healthcare practitioners and get helpful advice about coping with any uncomfortable symptoms. Besides, at most visits, a mom-to-be gets to listen to the beat of her baby's heart (an exciting and reassuring sound) and maybe even catch a glimpse of her child-to-be on an ultrasound screen.

The first prenatal visit
Here's what to expect at—and bring to—your first prenatal visit:

- **Physical examination.** You will have a full physical examination, including a pelvic exam and, if you have not had one in the past year, a Pap test. Pelvic

Q: Between hearing a heartbeat early in pregnancy and feeling the first kick months later, how can I tell if my baby's development is going well?

A: I know that the big block of time between these two milestones can cause a lot of anxiety, especially for a first-time mom, who may not feel that first welcome kick for a full 22 weeks. Most mothers-to-be get some reassurance from hearing their baby's heartbeat at their regular prenatal visits. During these visits, your healthcare practitioner also looks for other signs that all is well with mother and child as he asks you about how you are feeling, monitors your weight gain, measures your growing abdomen, and runs other checks. If anything seems unusual, he can perform additional procedures, such as ultrasounds and blood tests, to evaluate the situation, and, with any luck, give you some peace of mind.

exams usually include checking for inflammation or lesions on the genitalia, inspecting the condition of the vagina and cervix, and feeling for any abnormalities of the ovaries or uterus.

• **Medical history.** You and the baby's father will be asked about your medical, family, and reproductive health histories. If the dad can't be there, be sure to ask him about his medical history before the appointment. This is critical because it will help your practitioner anticipate—and sometimes prevent— problems that might arise for you or your baby. For example, diabetes, epilepsy, depression, or heart problems may complicate pregnancy.

- **Laboratory tests**. Routine tests include blood typing, a check for immunity to rubella (German measles), a blood count, and a urine culture. The blood typing will determine if you're type A, B, AB, or O, and if you're Rh-negative or -positive (problems may arise if you're Rh-negative and the fetus is Rh-positive; see page 149). It's important to check for immunity to rubella because contracting this disease while you're pregnant could lead to serious complications for the baby. If you don't have immunity, you'll have to be diligent to avoid possible sources of infection, and you can get vaccinated after the baby is born. The blood count indicates if you're anemic or have a low platelet count, which can affect blood clotting. The urine culture looks for evidence of a urinary tract infection (see page 72). In addition, even if you are at low risk for sexually transmitted infections, your practitioner will test your cervix for chlamydia and gonorrhea and your blood for hepatitis B and syphilis. If you are of African descent, you will be tested for sickle cell trait. All pregnant women should be offered HIV testing.

- **Due date.** Your practitioner will calculate your due date at this visit (see page 24). Bring all the information that might be helpful: your menstrual record, including the date of your last period; when you did any home pregnancy tests; records if you happened to perform ovulation detection or took basal body temperatures; and the date of conception, if known. If you're not sure when your last period was or when you conceived, your practitioner can calculate your due date using ultrasound (see page 48).

- **Risk assessment.** In addition to medical, reproductive, and family histories, your practitioner will probably ask about your diet; medication use; exposure to drugs, alcohol, or cigarettes; and personal and social issues.

- **Genetic concerns.** Bring along a copy of your and the father's family trees if you can, noting the regions of the world your ancestors came from and any known medical problems immediate family members have had (cystic fibrosis, sickle cell disease or trait, mental retardation, congenital heart diseases, etc.). Depending on your situation, your practitioner may refer you to a specialist for genetic testing or counseling (see page 26).

- **Nutritional counseling.** Women who are overweight, and particularly women who are underweight or who have eating disorders, must pay special attention to their nutritional needs in pregnancy. Vegetarians, especially vegans, need to be careful that they're getting adequate protein and vitamins. If you have special concerns, this is a good time to see a dietitian. Also, let your practitioner know if you take vitamin or nutritional supplements, as some of these can be toxic in pregnancy.

ULTRASOUND IN THE FIRST TRIMESTER

Ultrasound is a method of creating an image by "bouncing" sound waves off tissues. The current technology uses real-time ultrasound, meaning that you see pictures on a screen as they are obtained. These images also can be recorded digitally, on videotape, or in still photos (see page 126). While some doctors perform these scans routinely in the first trimester, most practitioners reserve early ultrasounds for special situations— for instance, when a woman has had some bleeding, when there's a risk for an ectopic pregnancy (see page 41), or to assess the size of the fetus if the due date is uncertain. Early ultrasounds also can be used to look for twins or other multiples.

When early ultrasound fails to detect the pregnancy in the uterus, it often means that a miscarriage has occurred; a doctor usually will run serial blood hCG tests (see page 97) or follow up with another ultrasound a few days later to be sure. In some cases, however, it could just be that the embryo is still too small to see. One thing first-trimester ultrasounds can't do that later ultrasounds can is help determine the sex of the baby; it is too early to see much in the way of the fetal anatomy, including the genitals.

LOOKING AHEAD

Your pregnancy may feel very real to you right now, but reactions to this life-changing event often kick in later with dads-to-be. Like you, your spouse or partner is sure to be subject to a roller-coaster ride of emotions, feeling proud and confident one moment, full of doubts and fears the next. Pregnancy is a time when prior problems in the relationship may be amplified, and these additional conflicts and stresses need to be worked out. But it is also a wonderful opportunity for your relationship to grow, as you both may be keenly motivated to work on communication. After all, you're embarking on a most amazing venture together.

Getting the dad-to-be involved

Many men feel that they are not included in the pregnancy experiences—that, for better or worse, it is a woman's world. But the more your spouse or partner understands about what both of you are going through, the better prepared and more supportive he can be. In fact, some men get so caught up in the pregnancy that they even experience physical symptoms, such as nausea or weight gain, right along with the mom-to-be. Besides, the earlier your partner gets involved in the whole pregnancy process, the more likely he'll be to stay that way when he actually becomes a dad.

One good way to get your spouse or partner involved is to go to prenatal visits together. This is a time for both of you to get to know your doctor or midwife, and to discuss your ideas and preferences for your baby's birth. In addition, a father-to-be gets to ask his own questions and

listen firsthand to what the healthcare practitioner recommends. Having the dad present is particularly valuable for a pre-conception appointment, the first prenatal
visit, the visits around the time of genetic screenings, and
if problems are developing in the pregnancy. Any
appointment in which an ultrasound is scheduled is also
a great chance for the father to bond with his baby-to-be.

Pregnancy changes your sex life

Whether sex is better than before, slightly uncomfortable, or completely absent, virtually every couple dis-
covers that their sexual relationship changes in some
way during the course of pregnancy. While some couples find that sexual desire is enhanced during this
time, others find it lacking. There are many reasons
why this might occur, including:

- **Concern for the baby.** Both the mother- and the
  father-to-be may worry that making love might
  injure the baby in some way or cause a miscarriage.
  This fear keeps them from enjoying the activity that
  got them pregnant in the first place. It might be
  helpful to know that the fetus is protected inside
  your uterus by the amniotic sac. Keep in mind that
  sex is perfectly safe in normal, low-risk pregnancies,
  so try not to let unfounded medical concerns limit
  your ability to relax and enjoy.

- **Cramping and bleeding.** A number of women worry
  about any cramping that they might experience during or after intercourse. Semen in the vagina, sexual
  arousal, and orgasm can all cause the uterus to

cramp. This is normal. The cramping should subside soon after intercourse. Occasionally, a woman will experience vaginal spotting after intercourse in the first trimester. If this happens to you, refrain from having intercourse again until you discuss with your practitioner the need for any possible restrictions on your sex life. Generally, couples are advised to avoid intercourse until the bleeding has resolved and the pregnancy has been shown (by physical examination or ultrasound) to be progressing normally. If bleeding is heavy and is accompanied by severe cramps or lasts more than a few hours, call your practitioner.

PARENT TO PARENT

"I believe that some men are really in tune with what their partner is feeling during pregnancy. I personally know a few couples where the fathers swore that they went through morning sickness with the mothers."

—**kelly225,** AS POSTED ON DRSPOCK.COM

• **Mom's attitude toward sex.** Many women have less interest in sex during the first trimester. Let's face it: It's hard to feel frisky when you're completely exhausted, your breasts feel like pincushions, and you can't stop throwing up! But if they're spared from such symptoms, some pregnant women find that they experience better sex than ever before. This could be because of changing hormones or because they have never felt closer to their partners or so carefree about birth control. And for women who have gone through fertility treatment, the relationship between sex and the pressure to conceive is over. They certainly don't need to worry about it now!

• **Dad's attitude toward sex.** Some men find their pregnant wives sexier than ever. They may be excited by the physical changes in their partners, may feel especially close to them emotionally, and may even be a bit proud to show off this proof of their own masculinity. Other men, however, find pregnancy a bit of a sexual turnoff or begrudge the fact that their partner's body is now dedicated to a function other than their own physical pleasure. If you sense that your spouse or partner is less than thrilled by your pregnancy, try to get him to talk about his feelings—and try to listen openly, without passing judgment, even if you're disappointed by his reactions. This isn't always easy, I know, but you'll do your relationship a world of good if you can understand where your spouse is coming from and provide him the reassurance—or space—that he needs. Remember that even men who seem reluctant to embrace their wives' pregnancies at first often become excited about the prospect of becoming a father later on. And don't hesitate to seek help from a marital therapist or other counselor if you two can't seem to work through any problems on your own: Lots of couples go through a rough patch, especially with first pregnancies.

CONDOMS IN PREGNANCY

In general, it's safe to have sex throughout pregnancy until your water breaks (see page 238) or you are in active labor. However, if you or your partner has other sexual partners, or if just one of you has herpes or genital warts, be sure to use condoms to prevent transmitting infection. If you aren't sure if condoms are necessary, discuss your situation with your healthcare practitioner.

NOTES

Use this space to jot down observations about your pregnancy or questions to ask your healthcare practitioner at your next visit:

_____

_____

_____

_____

_____

_____

_____

_____

_____

_____

_____

_____

CHAPTER 3

Weeks 9–13

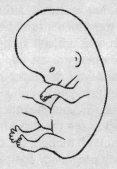

At 10 weeks, your baby is curled into a ball measuring about 1¼ inches from crown to rump, and weighing about ⅓ ounce. By Week 11, all of the main organ systems are in place.

ABOUT YOUR BABY

Up until about the 10th week of gestation, the developing wonder inside you is formally referred to as an "embryo" as far as the medical world is concerned. After the 10-week milestone, however, it is officially dubbed a "fetus." (And you've probably been thinking about it all along simply as your "baby.") Many of the most dramatic transformations have already taken place: Inside your little bundle, intestines, liver, kidneys, lungs, and heart are all well under way, and, depending on the child's sex, either the ovaries or the testes have formed. But there is still a lot of development that needs to take place before your baby is ready to emerge into the world.

By Week 10, your baby is starting to make tiny movements with her muscles, although you won't begin to feel her movements until between 16 and 22 weeks. It is sometimes difficult to get through these next few months, when you are hoping all is OK with your pregnancy and you don't yet have your baby's movements to constantly reassure you. Once you hear the fetal heartbeat in your healthcare practitioner's office (see page 74) or see the flickering of the beating heart on an ultrasound, though, the chance of miscarriage or other early pregnancy complication goes way down, and you can relax and enjoy.

ABOUT YOU

In the third month, your uterus grows to the size of a navel orange. You may still fit in your regular clothes, but you are likely to be choosing the loosest ones in the bunch and avoiding those skinny jeans. Many mothers-to-be buy (or borrow) some soft, stretchy non-maternity clothes about this time, trying to get through the next couple of months without having to don real maternity clothing. Hold on to these outfits when you outgrow them—they also will serve you well in the first few months after the baby arrives.

By the end of the third month, you may start feeling

a little better, regaining a bit more of your former energy and experiencing less nausea. Now that your symptoms are less distracting, you may be ready to think of enjoying your life during pregnancy instead of feeling taken over by your symptoms—a very common phenomenon in early pregnancy.

Moms-to-be need exercise

Every day, it seems, a new study comes out proving that regular exercise has tremendous health benefits, from warding off stroke and heart disease to keeping the body lean and the mind keen. And while some women, particularly those experiencing a high-risk pregnancy, may be better off avoiding strenuous activity, most moms-to-be can participate safely in vigorous exercise, even if they weren't active before pregnancy. Exercise is good for your mood, for weight control, and for strength and stamina. Women who exercise regularly during pregnancy tend to have shorter labors and slightly thinner babies (which, later in life, may help them stay trim, since chubby babies are prone to become overweight adults). But before joining a gym or lacing up your running shoes, be sure to discuss any exercise plans with your healthcare practitioner to make be sure that the activities are safe for your individual situation.

So what's safe—and what's not?

Swimming or participating in water aerobics is probably the best type of exercise for pregnant women. The water supports your extra weight, helps you stay cool, lessens any swelling in your legs, and generally makes you feel refreshed and invigorated. Snorkeling is also safe in pregnancy.

If you prefer to take your exercise on terra firma, however, walking and low-impact aerobics are good ways to go. While special classes for pregnant women are great (not only are the routines tailored to your needs, but it's fun to be in a class full of other expectant moms!), regular low-impact aerobic classes are generally fine as well. The use of aerobic-exercise machines such as stair-steppers, treadmills, stationary bicycles, and ski machines is OK, as long as you follow the principles for safe exercise in pregnancy (see page 59). Cross-country skiing, jogging, and tennis are fine for women who already are regular participants in these sports and are confident that they can avoid falls or injuries. If you're experienced and willing to take it easy, horseback riding, ice skating, in-line skating, and downhill skiing (at low altitudes) are somewhat riskier but probably still reasonable activities.

No matter how experienced you are, however, there are certain activities that you really should avoid when you're pregnant. Save the waterskiing until after your baby is born: There have been rare reports of injuries to the birth canal in waterskiing accidents. Skiing at high altitudes and scuba diving are probably not safe for the fetus and therefore should be avoided. The first poses the risk of a compromised oxygen supply, and the second can result in a case of the bends for the fetus.

Principles for safe exercise

1. Exercise is good.

Thirty minutes of moderate exercise every day is an excellent goal for pregnant women. (It's not bad for non-pregnant folks, either!) Don't push yourself too hard: You should feel as if you're working hard but could still hold a conversation. Going for a brisk walk (about a three-to-four-mile-per-hour pace) for about 30 minutes every day is a great start for those who aren't used to exercising regularly.

2. Listen to your body.
If you feel dizzy, light-headed, or short of breath, you should rest. Once you feel better, you can resume your activities at a slower pace.

3. Avoid getting overheated.
Raising your body temperature is not good for the baby. Dress appropriately for the activity and slow down or stop if you feel that you're getting overheated.

4. Keep well hydrated.
Carry a water bottle with you, and pause frequently for a drink.

5. Stay off your back.
Avoid exercises that keep you flat on your back for more than a few minutes at a time (this is especially important after your fifth month of pregnancy). The weight of your uterus can decrease blood flow through the large veins that lie behind it. This can compromise oxygen delivery to your developing baby and can make you feel woozy.

6. Avoid injury.
Your joints may be less stable due to the softening effects the pregnancy hormone progesterone has on your ligaments. As an added challenge, your center of gravity moves forward as the baby grows, throwing off your sense of balance. Although the baby is well cushioned in his amniotic sac, avoid activities in which you are likely to fall or hit your abdomen.

Protect your back by being careful about lifting

Although your baby is protected in your uterus and won't be hurt, lifting heavy objects can put stress on your back and lead to intermittent or chronic back pain. Doctors are divided about how much weight is safe for a pregnant woman to lift, so if you are concerned about your back or have to do heavy lifting at your job, be sure to discuss weight limits with your own healthcare practitioner.

To minimize the chances of hurting yourself while lifting something heavy:

- **Lift from your legs.** Squat down and use your legs to bear much of the weight as you stand up.
- **Don't lean over.** Bending over as you lift puts all the stress of the weight on your back.
- **Ask someone to help.** Back pain in pregnancy is common enough without bringing it on yourself. This is no time to be proud: Ask for help whenever possible—particularly if you already have been experiencing back pain.
- **Let your children climb up onto you.** It may be impossible, especially if you have a toddler, to avoid lifting and carrying your child periodically. No doubt there will be times when you need to immediately rescue him from an unsafe situation or when he just needs you to hold him. As much as possible, have your child climb up onto your lap for a snuggle instead of picking him up from the floor. Your back will thank you. (See Chapter 7 for more information on safe lifting and back pain in later pregnancy.)

Treating routine illnesses isn't routine in pregnancy

In the normal course of events, there are many symptoms and illnesses that most of us treat on our own.

But when you're expecting, dealing with a cold or a nagging headache becomes a bit more complicated— after all, now you have your developing baby's health to think about as well.

If you become ill during your pregnancy, first be sure that you don't have a serious problem. In general, coughs and colds are not dangerous conditions. They may be annoying and make you feel awful, but neither presents a real risk to your health or the health of your baby. If you are ill for more than a few days, develop a high fever, have a severe sore throat or headache (see page 65), or are worried that your symptoms seem unusual, you should see your healthcare practitioner. When you're treating yourself, try to start with non-medical measures. For example, if you have a cough or cold, you can:

- **Drink plenty of fluids.** This helps thin secretions. Water, chicken soup, juices, and warm, noncaffeinated tea are good choices.
- **Use a humidifier.** Place it close to your face when you sleep. During the day, you can make a tent out of a towel draped over your head as you stand above your vaporizer or the sink with the hot water running. Taking a warm shower also can help loosen secretions and soothe aching muscles.
- **Use menthol.** Rub a mentholated product (like Vicks VapoRub) on your chest or put a dab under your nose if you are congested.

- **Elevate your head when you sleep.** To make breathing easier, sleep in a recliner or prop up your head with a few pillows so that you are in a semiupright position.
- **Get plenty of rest.** You probably won't feel like doing much anyway.

COUGHING AND INCONTINENCE 🐾

If you develop a severe cough, rest assured that the fetus is protected inside your uterus: You can't cough so hard that you miscarry or go into labor. However, it's not uncommon to experience some leakage of urine during a coughing or sneezing fit. Probably the best thing you can do about stress urinary incontinence is to empty your bladder frequently and practice your Kegel (or pelvic-floor muscle) exercises (see page 196).

Some OTC medications are safer than others

While it is generally best to avoid exposing a fetus to medications, especially in the first trimester, when the organs are forming, sometimes drugs are necessary either for medical reasons or for relieving severe symptoms. Here are some common over-the-counter (OTC) medications that are probably safe during pregnancy (see page 75 for information on prescription medications):

- **Decongestants.** This group of medications is used to treat colds or allergies. Pseudoephedrine is present in many OTC allergy and cold remedies, such as Sudafed. These medications are *not* recommended for anyone who has high blood pressure. If possible, avoid taking pseudoephedrine in the first trimester.

- **Cough suppressants and expectorants**. Dextromethorphan, a common ingredient found in cough and cold medications (such as Robitussin), is probably safe for use in pregnancy. Guaifenesin is an expectorant found in many cough and cold medicines, and also seems to be OK. Unless you're diabetic, an even safer alternative is to try a mixture of honey (to soothe the tickle) and lemon juice (to help clear the phlegm). You can use any proportions of the two ingredients, and you can take the mixture as often as you like.

- **Treating pain and fever.** Fever is bad because it overheats the fetus. This is unhealthy throughout pregnancy and is especially dangerous in the first trimester, when high fever is thought to be responsible for certain birth defects, including problems in brain and spine development. It's generally best to follow this rule: If you get a fever in pregnancy, take medications to bring it down, and if you cannot reduce your temperature, call your doctor.

  Whether they're dealing with fever or pain, most pregnant women can take acetaminophen (Tylenol) without a problem. If you are a heavy drinker (three or more drinks a day), you need to talk with your practitioner, not only because drinking while pregnant has health implications for your baby (see page 10), but because alcohol and acetaminophen can be a lethal combination. Ibuprofen (Motrin, Advil) is probably safe to take in the first and second trimesters, but it may cause problems for the baby's circulation after 32 weeks' gestation. Aspirin is usually not recommended for fever or pain in pregnancy.

Remember: A persistent fever or severe illness in pregnancy always warrants a call to your healthcare practitioner.

Treat headaches step by step

Because headaches are so common, I want to provide you with more specific information about how to treat them while you're pregnant.

First, keep in mind that prevention is always better than treatment. If you know what seems to bring on your headaches, plan ahead and avoid triggers. A lack of sleep, low blood sugar (which may affect pregnant women who eat irregularly), alcohol use, and loud noises (such as encountered at rock concerts) all can set off tension headaches or migraines. Migraine headaches are also more common in smokers—yet one more reason to quit.

Second, use a stepwise approach to treatment:

- **Nonmedical treatment for pain.** Applying a cool compress to your forehead, resting in a cool dark room, taking a nap, gently massaging your temples, or getting a massage may make you feel better without the use of medications. You also can try meditating, relaxation techniques, soothing music, or an ice pack for your head or face.

- **Non-narcotic pain medications.** Acetaminophen (Tylenol) is the usual first-line treatment for pain in pregnancy. Before the third trimester, nonsteroidals like ibuprofen (Motrin, Advil) are generally considered safe. After 32 weeks, potential adverse effects on the fetus's circulation and kidney function limit the safe use of this class of drugs. One cup of coffee or a caffeinated soft drink a day is usually considered safe at any stage of pregnancy and may help the headache. It is a good idea to use nonmedical treatments in addition to pain medications, and to try to limit the amount of medication you take, especially in the first trimester.

- **Narcotic pain medications.** If the first-line pain therapies don't work, sometimes narcotic pain medications like codeine, oxycodone (Percodan), and meperidine (Demerol) are prescribed for severe headache in pregnancy. While this type of medication is addictive if used for long stretches of time (weeks or more), short-term use poses surprisingly little risk to mother or fetus as long as the mother doesn't drive or operate heavy machinery. These are prescription medications that, of course, are taken only in consultation with your OB practitioner. When pain is severe, intravenous or injectable pain medications may be necessary for the mother's well-being. Nausea medication such as prochlorperazine (Compazine) also may help.

- **Dealing with migraines.** Prescription migraine drugs are recommended as a last resort, mostly because healthcare professionals don't have long-term experience with their patients' using them during pregnancy. Some migraine medications (such as ergotamine, found in Cafergot) are definitely not safe in pregnancy, so be sure to check with your practitioner before using your usual migraine meds.

WARNING SIGNS THAT A HEADACHE NEEDS URGENT EVALUATION BY A PHYSICIAN

- It is different from any headache you have had before.
- It is severe and occurs immediately upon waking in the morning or disturbs your sleep.
- It is accompanied by vision problems, or numbness or weakness in a limb.
- You are already being monitored for high blood pressure and the pain doesn't respond to acetaminophen.

Be prepared to deal with stress

There are numerous reports of stress leading to serious complications during pregnancy. You can't prevent bad things from happening, of course, and you can't suddenly change your emotional responses. But you can

Q: I just found out that I'm pregnant. I know that I'm supposed to stay away from caffeine, but I'm a three-cup-a-day coffee drinker. Is there any way to avoid caffeine-withdrawal headaches? I've gotten them before, and they're nasty!

A: Many women give up caffeine suddenly when they learn that they're pregnant, only to find themselves experiencing headaches for several days as their bodies adjust to withdrawal. Small amounts of caffeine, like that found in one cup of coffee or soft drink, haven't been shown to harm the fetus, so it may be reasonable to cut down over a few days rather than quitting cold turkey. Sometimes just realizing that the headache is caused by caffeine withdrawal is reassuring, since you know that it's not something more serious and that you'll have to tolerate only a few days of discomfort.

use stress management techniques to protect yourself (and perhaps your baby) from some of stress's negative effects.

As you probably know, your emotional state can cause physical changes in your body, such as a quickening heart rate and an elevation in the level of stress hormones. These, in turn, can affect your baby. And if you feel upset or sad and deal with it by smoking, drinking alcohol, eating poorly, or not sleeping, these responses, too, can have a negative effect on your pregnancy.

If you're feeling depressed, overwhelmed, or generally stressed out during your pregnancy, try to take decisive action quickly. For example:

- **Get support.** Social isolation is one of the factors that can intensify stress and depression. Talk to your family and friends, join a support group, get counseling from a therapist or member of the clergy, or connect with an Internet community in chat rooms or on message boards. While it may seem impossible to feel happier when you're experiencing difficult times, reaching out to others can minimize feelings of isolation.

- **Participate in activities that lower stress.** Meditation, yoga, music, and massage all can help you manage stress. There is ample evidence that these activities actually can affect your physical responses to anxiety, such as lowering heart-rate and stress-hormone levels.

- **Eat a healthy diet.** Fresh fruits, vegetables, and whole grains are among the best foods you can eat during pregnancy—or anytime, for that matter. If you know you aren't eating well, be sure to at least take a multivitamin and talk to your healthcare practitioner about what else you should do.

- **Get plenty of exercise.** Lots of studies have demonstrated the benefits of exercise during pregnancy, for both physical and mental health (see page 57).

Just be sure to check with your practitioner before you start any kind of exercise program.

- **Don't take risks.** I'm not talking about the obvious here, like heading out to scale Mount McKinley. If you find that you are driving in an unsafe way because you are distracted or are crying too hard, pull over. Emotional events sometimes can have as much effect on your reflexes as alcohol, or as the strong medications that you should avoid while driving or operating heavy machinery. Also, you might want to postpone any major, life-changing decisions until you feel more like yourself.

- **Avoid unhealthy habits that serve as emotional crutches.** Seek out alternative activities if you are craving cigarettes or alcohol. Try exercise, talking to a friend, singing, eating carrots, chewing gum, crying—whatever works for you.

All of us get blue or stressed out at some time or another, and you don't have to worry about the normal ups and downs of living putting your baby at risk. However, you should seek professional assistance if you are thinking about harming yourself or others, if you are still unable to function in your daily activities after a few days have passed, if your feelings frighten you, or if your loved ones are telling you that they are worried about you. There are safe medications that can provide temporary relief from severe anxiety and depression. If you think you are reaching the point where it might be necessary to take such medication, talk to your practitioner or see a psychotherapist or psychiatrist.

GETTING GOOD CARE

For most of history, pregnant women received health advice from family, friends, and midwives. It's only in the last century that a regular schedule of prenatal care from doctors was added to the mix. Initially, the purpose of this professional prenatal care was to identify moms-to-be who were developing high blood pressure in the third trimester. The visits then were expanded to include screening for risk factors early in pregnancy, establishing a clear due date, and watching for signs of other developing problems. Now prenatal care often includes counseling about diet and lifestyle, sorting out normal symptoms from worrisome ones, and education about what to expect in the course of pregnancy and birth.

Prenatal appointments will become part of your routine

The first prenatal visit will usually be the longest, and you will have the most complete physical examination (see page 44). Subsequent prenatal visits are usually scheduled at four-week intervals through the seventh month, then at two-week intervals, and, finally, weekly in the last month. Your practitioner may need to see you less often if you are at low risk, more often if potential problems are developing.

At these routine visits, the medical staff will check your blood pressure, weight, and urine. Your practitioner will also do a "tummy check" to see how the baby is growing and listen to the fetal heartbeat. Internal exams usually aren't done until later in pregnancy unless you have certain risk factors or exhibit signs of developing problems. Your practitioner will ask you about any problems you may be experiencing, so be sure to report how you are feeling, and don't hesitate to ask lots of questions.

So, what are they looking for in your urine, anyway?

At every prenatal visit, your urine is tested for protein and glucose (sugar). This can give your practitioner a hint of whether or not you are developing diabetes of pregnancy (see page 147) or preeclampsia (see page 231). Sometimes protein in the urine also can be a sign of a urinary tract infection, or UTI. Urine culture for infection is done at the first visit, and again later if you have any signs of infection such as discomfort with urination. Urinating frequently and leaking a little urine with a cough or sneeze is normal in pregnancy.

Urinary tract infections are among the most common medical problems that expectant mothers face. Between two and seven percent of pregnant women will have urine cultures that test positive for bacteria, and even without these tests, some women would recognize that they have a UTI because of the familiar symptoms: a need to urinate frequently, a burning sensation while urinating, discomfort after voiding, and, sometimes, blood in the urine. However, most pregnant women with UTIs have none of the classic symptoms—thus, the routine screenings to catch the infections. The bacteria that cause urinary tract infections usually come from your own body: They live in the intestinal tract or the skin near the opening of the bladder. Your doctor can prescribe an antibiotic that is known to be safe in pregnancy to quickly cure the infection.

It is very important to receive treatment for UTIs. Mild infections, which can be asymptomatic (without obvious symptoms), can turn into severe ones, with plenty of pain for you and consequences for the baby, including preterm uterine contractions.

Kidney infections can be hard to diagnose

When doctors use the term UTI, they're usually referring to an infection of the lower urinary tract. Much more rare but caused by the same bacteria are upper urinary tract infections, commonly called kidney infections or pyelonephritis. Although they typically don't cause the telltale bladder symptoms that alert some women to the presence of UTIs, these more serious infections often are accompanied by fever, chills, and back or side pain. In addition, some people experience nausea and vomiting, leading them to suspect food poisoning or appendicitis instead of the real culprit. If you develop any of the symptoms mentioned above, you need to see your doctor right away—even if it's after office hours. Kidney infections can lead to premature labor, bacteria in the bloodstream (blood poisoning), and difficulty breathing. Treatment usually involves intravenous antibiotics in the hospital until the fever subsides and the possibility of serious complications has passed.

Doppler instruments let you listen to your baby's heartbeat

By the 9th or 10th week after your last menstrual period, you might be able to hear your baby's heartbeat at your prenatal appointment. Your obstetrical practitioner probably uses a Doppler instrument for this purpose, which bounces harmless sound waves off the fetal heart. The way the sound comes back is affected by motion, so a beating heart creates a change in the sound that can be picked up by the receiver in the Doppler. Whether you actually hear the heartbeat at this early stage depends partly on luck: The instrument must be placed at just the right angle. It also depends on the position of your uterus, and if you're slim or heavy. By the 12th week, the heartbeat can usually be heard consistently, using the Doppler instrument for amplification.

PARENT TO PARENT

"Hi, everyone! I wanted to share with you that we finally heard the baby's heartbeat today. Even though I am still nauseous (a little less each day), listening to the baby's heartbeat was just what I needed."

—**babywood**, AS POSTED ON DRSPOCK.COM

Your doctor will measure the fetal heart rate

To determine the baby's heart rate, your practitioner may count the heartbeats for a full minute, or count for 15 seconds and then multiply by four. Some instruments eliminate the need for this by providing a readout of the rate. And some practitioners are so attuned to the normal range that they listen carefully and count only if the heart rate seems high or low.

At times, the Doppler picks up sounds from the mother's side of the placenta and relays her heartbeat instead of the fetus's. A normal heart rate for the mother is under 100, but the baby's should be over 120, so they sound different. If there is a question, the practitioner will feel the mother's pulse and see if it's the same as what she's listening to through the Doppler instrument.

A normal fetal heart rate usually is between 120 and 160 beats per minute. While rumors abound about using the heart rate to tell if a baby is a girl or a boy, there is a lot of overlap between girls' and boys' rates, so this isn't a reliable method to choose baby clothes or room decor. The loudness or quietness of the heartbeat also doesn't mean anything. The sound has to do only with the volume controls on the instrument as well as the distance and angle from the heart to the Doppler. So don't worry if it sounds quiet or far away sometimes.

Some prescription medications are fine during pregnancy

Earlier in this chapter, I went over some of the OTC medications that are safe to take during pregnancy for common problems such as coughs, colds, and headaches. Now I'd like to discuss some of the issues involving prescription medicines and pregnancy, a topic that my own obstetrical patients often ask about during their office visits.

These questions actually aren't that easy to answer. In order to say that a drug is safe, researchers must compare the babies of women who took this medicine to the babies of women who did everything else exactly the same except for taking that particular drug. But pregnant women don't often volunteer for research studies to see if a medicine is safe for the fetus, and no two women are exactly alike. So most of the time, we look at research done on pregnant animals—and on data from women who happened to take that medication—to try to guess if the drug will cause any problems.

However, there are a few medications that have been tested in pregnant human subjects and have been shown to be safe. Examples include folic acid and vitamin B_6 (both in the B vitamin family) and levothyroxine (Synthroid), which replaces the thyroid hormone in people whose glands aren't functioning. These are known by the FDA as **Category A** medications.

Most medications, though, have not been studied or shown to be safe to this extent. Medications that are considered relatively safe to use in pregnancy are those that have been used for many years and don't *appear* to cause any major birth defects or other problems. (They also have been shown not to cause birth defects in animals.) The FDA classifies these drugs as **Category B.** This group includes ampicillin, acetaminophen

(Tylenol is a common brand), aspartame, caffeine in moderation, heparin, metoclopramide (Reglan), famotidine (Pepcid), prednisone, insulin, and, before the third trimester, ibuprofen (such as Motrin).

Category C medications are somewhat more likely to cause some complications for mother or fetus, or there isn't enough research to draw conclusions about their safety. These medications come with the warning that they should be used only if the potential benefits outweigh the possible risks. These include prochlorperazine (Compazine), albuterol (Ventolin), fluconazole (Diflucan), and ciprofloxacin (Cipro). In fact, most prescription medications are classified in Category C.

Category D medications are those that clearly have health risks for the fetus, including ethanol (alcohol), lithium, phenytoin (Dilantin), and most chemotherapy agents. These still may be used under certain circumstances.

Category X drugs have been shown to cause birth defects and are not to be used in pregnancy under any circumstances. This category includes isotretinoin (Accutane), thalidomide, and diethylstilbestrol (DES).

LOOKING AHEAD

Some couples shout their good news from the rooftops as soon as they have a positive pregnancy test, while others want to wait until they are several months along. By the end of the first trimester, if you have heard a fetal heartbeat in your practitioner's office or seen one on ultrasound, your chance of miscarriage is under 1 percent. If you haven't already told everyone you know, it is probably time to share your glad tidings with friends and family. After all, a pregnancy is a real milestone in your life. Sharing the word that a new family member is on the way leads to joyous and meaningful moments that you don't want to miss.

In your excitement, though, it's easy to forget the effect that the announcement of your pregnancy may have on others. Perhaps some of your friends or family members have had a miscarriage or lost a child, while others may be having difficulty conceiving. Although they're sure to be happy for you, the news of your good fortune may accentuate their own sadness and frustration. Be prepared to hear these mixed feelings, and don't take them personally. It may be a tough time for your relationship, but good communication and sensitivity to each other's feelings can help keep the air clear.

When it comes to pregnancy, big is beautiful
By now, you've already started to gain a little extra weight; most women gain at least a few pounds by the end of their first trimester. This probably doesn't bother you, but as the months go by and the pounds keep packing on, you may start seeing the scale as your new worst enemy.

This reaction is completely understandable in our culture. Many American women spend much of their lives struggling to lose weight or avoid extra pounds.

No wonder that it's sometimes hard for women to allow themselves to gain appropriately for a pregnancy! But as your pregnancy progresses, it is important to remember that this weight gain is for a purpose: Your body is accomplishing a miracle, and it needs energy and nutrients to do it.

How much weight should you gain?

An ideal pregnancy weight gain starts with the addition of 7 to 10 pounds in the first 20 weeks of pregnancy. Subsequently, during the second half of the pregnancy, you would gain around a half pound to a pound each week. All told, current guidelines recommend that an average-size woman should gain somewhere between 25 and 35 pounds during her pregnancy. If a woman already was overweight when she became pregnant, most experts suggest that she gain between 15 and 20 pounds. Your healthcare professional can help determine the appropriate weight gain in your particular case.

Don't use pregnancy as an excuse to eat, and, conversely, don't go crazy worrying that you're racking up the pounds. The main objective is to consume a healthy, well-balanced diet based on a variety of foods (see page 38). A woman who is *not* pregnant needs between 1,800 and 2,200 calories per day. When you are pregnant, you need to take in an additional 300 or so calories per day. You will probably gain the right amount of weight if you generally eat healthy foods and let your own appetite be your guide.

What if you gain too much or too little?

The amount of weight you gain is important. Although many women worry that they are gaining too much, your practitioner will probably be more concerned if you are not gaining enough. Poor weight gain increases the chances that the baby will not get adequate nutrition or grow properly. Sometimes eating more frequently (adding additional small meals or healthy snacks) and increasing the fat in your diet can help.

Excess weight gain is not usually a medical problem. The biggest negative about gaining too much weight is

---

THE DISTRIBUTION OF PREGNANCY POUNDS: WHAT GOES WHERE?

Wondering where all those extra pounds are going? Here's how the weight gain is distributed in a typical pregnancy:

Baby: 7 pounds
Placenta: 1 pound
Amniotic fluid: 2 pounds
Blood volume: 4 pounds
Body fluids: 3 pounds
Uterus: 2 pounds
Breasts: 1 pound
Fat and protein storage: 7 pounds

that it may be depressing to contemplate trying to lose those pounds after the baby is born. If you are gaining weight too quickly, you still need to eat when you're hungry, but try to decrease your portion size, eat more slowly, and substitute lower-fat foods for higher (such as skim milk instead of 2 percent, and frozen yogurt instead of ice cream). Rapid weight gain, more than four pounds in a week, can be a sign of severe fluid retention from preeclampsia if your blood pressure is also high. If you are worried about your weight gain or diet, discuss your concerns with your doctor or midwife. Sometimes a consultation with a dietitian also can be helpful.

When twins are on board, special circumstances apply

If you are carrying twins (see page 87) or other multiples, of course, you should gain more weight. Your physician will discuss your ideal weight gain with you. With twins, for example, the typical optimal weight gain is between 35 and 45 pounds.

PARENT TO PARENT

"I am 24 and very overweight. I am really worried that I won't be able to feel the baby like women who are average weight. I am worried that I won't have enough energy to push the baby out. I will always regret not losing weight before I got pregnant, but that's my goal next time around <lol!>. Can anyone give me any advice?"

—**hunniebear,** AS POSTED ON DRSPOCK.COM

"I work in the labor and delivery ward, and I can tell you that there are many women out there on the 'larger' side who give birth to healthy babies every day! Focus on your baby and, yes, you will feel the kicks and movement! Delivery should be fine—you'll be able to do things you never thought you could do that day! Good luck and congrats!"

—**crimakian,** AS POSTED ON DRSPOCK.COM

NOTES

Use this space to jot down observations about your pregnancy or questions to ask your healthcare practitioner at your next visit:

_____

_____

_____

_____

_____

_____

_____

_____

_____

_____

_____

_____

_____

CHAPTER 4

Weeks 14—17

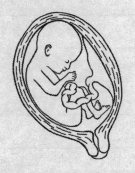

Your baby is now roughly about the size of your fist and weighs an ounce or so. The fetal organs continue to develop at a rapid pace, and if you could sneak a peek into the uterus, you could tell if your child is a boy or a girl.

ABOUT YOUR BABY

Welcome to the second trimester, usually a time of contentment and physical comfort for moms-to-be, no matter how rocky the first trimester. Your baby is now about 2¾ to 4 inches long, crown to rump, and weighs about an ounce. You may have felt him begin to stir, which is always an exciting time for expectant parents, and you probably have heard the sound of his heartbeat on a Doppler instrument in your OB's office. The intestines have formed, though they still need time to mature, and the pupils of your baby's eyes have developed, although his eyelids will be fused closed for another couple of months. He now has tiny fingernails, and the baby teeth that will emerge months after birth are starting to form in his jaws. In other words, your baby is looking more and more human.

Early in the pregnancy, the placenta produces amniotic fluid. During the fourth month or so, the baby's kidneys start to function and take over this job. Amniotic fluid, however, is not urine as we think of it. The majority of the baby's waste products actually are transported through the placenta into the mother's circulation and are then filtered by her kidneys. The baby does secrete some substances and shed fetal skin cells directly into the amniotic fluid, however. This is important because if amniocentesis needs to be performed, these substances in the fluid can provide clues to the fetus's condition (see page 94).

The baby's sex is now clear

No doubt you've been wondering if your baby will be a boy or a girl. A fetus destined to be a girl will have two X chromosomes, and a boy will have an X and a Y chromosome, but up until the eighth week of gestation, male and female genital systems are identical. As the baby matures, his or her genes will send out instructions that cause the gonads to become either ovaries or testicles, the phallus to become a

Q: I am in my second trimester. Although I am trying to sleep on my left side, I often wake up on my back and sometimes my stomach. Could this hurt the baby?

A: You are not alone in your concerns—it is difficult to follow rules while you are asleep! However, my belief is that most activities that are bad for you in pregnancy feel pretty terrible, which helps you not do them. If lying flat doesn't feel uncomfortable, it's probably OK for you to do so, at least right now. As you get bigger, however, it will be a good idea to avoid sleeping on your back. Lying flat on your back can cause the weight of the uterus to compress some big blood vessels running through the middle of your body. This can slow the flow of blood back to your heart and to the baby.

To help you sleep in the proper position, try placing a pillow under the right half of your back so that you are tipped a bit to the left. This tilted position is enough to prevent compression of the blood vessels. You also can lie all the way over on your right side with the same benefit, if that feels better to you.

clitoris or a penis, and the genital folds to turn into labia or a scrotum. By Week 12 to 14, while not fully formed, your baby's external genitalia are recognizably male or female. By Week 16 or so, if your baby is positioned in a favorable way, his or her sex can be identified during an ultrasound exam (see page 126). Before undergoing one, be sure to decide whether or not you want to know your baby's sex, and tell the ultrasound technician. Otherwise, she may spill the beans inadvertently!

Sometimes there's more than one baby on board

The fourth month is often the time that a couple finds out they are having twins or other multiples. While twins can be seen if ultrasound is done earlier in pregnancy, usually it is not until the fourth month of a twin pregnancy that the uterine size becomes noticeably bigger than normal. This early on, it is hard to distinguish the two separate heartbeats of twins during physical examination, so it is rare for your practitioner to be certain that there are twins before an ultrasound is done. For most expectant parents, the news that twins are on the way evokes a mixture of happy anticipation and apprehension. The parents are sure to have many questions, including speculation as to whether the pair will be identical or fraternal.

ABOUT YOU

In the fourth month, your uterus grows from about the size of a navel orange to the size of a really big grapefruit. Most mothers-to-be start to "show" this month, although some can hide their pregnancy with loose clothing, if they choose to. Generally, your energy level is good and your nausea is gone, or at least much improved.

IDENTICAL OR FRATERNAL TWINS? 🐣

In the United States today, about one-third of twins are identical. These pairs, with their breathtaking similarities, come from the same egg and sperm. Usually, after the egg and sperm have joined, the resultant cell, called a zygote, starts to multiply into the millions of diverse cells that eventually compose a single baby. In identical twins, however, the resultant cell separates into two zygotes, each with the same genetic material. This kind of twinning happens in about one out of every 240 pregnancies. It takes place among all families and cultures.

Fraternal twins, on the other hand, are the result of two different eggs becoming fertilized by two different sperm. Although both zygotes share the same uterus, they are no more similar than any other set of siblings. This kind of twinning runs in families and is prevalent in certain races. Africa sees the highest incidence of fraternal twins; Asia, the lowest. Fertility drugs increase your chances of having this type of pair.

Most of the time, parents have to wait until birth to find out if their twins are identical or fraternal. Occasionally, hints surface before then. For example, if the twins share the same amniotic sac, they are definitely identical, and this can be determined by ultrasound. However, the majority of identical twins, as well as all fraternal twins, have their own amniotic sac, so you still may be in the dark until the delivery. And, of course, if ultrasound determines one twin to be a girl and one to be a boy, you can be certain they are fraternal.

Women having a second (or subsequent) baby may start to feel movement by the end of this month, but first-time moms will have to wait a little longer. You also may start noticing a new set of physical changes to your body as you enter your second trimester, including dramatic changes to your skin, hair, and nails.

Hormones cause changes to your skin

During pregnancy, you may realize that you sunburn more easily, your skin gets unusually dry and itchy, or that you really do develop that special dewy glow that mothers-to-be are said to have. These are due to the hormones your body is producing. Here are some of the common problems—and benefits!—you may experience:

- **Your skin may break out more—or it may look better than ever.** Many women develop acne (or more severe acne) after they become pregnant. Try to keep your face as clean as possible, using a mild cleanser. If you wear makeup, be certain you use a water-based foundation. If you need to visit a dermatologist, inform her that you are pregnant. Some prescription medications she might normally prescribe are not safe during pregnancy. Conversely, other women who have had acne since adolescence find that their skin clears up during pregnancy.

- **You're likely to be more sensitive to the sun.** You'll probably find that you burn more easily, so lather on a good sunscreen (SPF 15 or higher), buy yourself a fetching wide-brimmed hat, and, in general, try to avoid the sun whenever you can. This is good advice even when you're not pregnant, since tanning increases the chance of skin cancer and causes wrinkles and age spots later in life. You may figure, Fine, if tanning is out, I'll just use one of those self-tanning products. But that's not a great idea, either. They haven't been proven to be safe for a developing fetus, and it's best to wait until after the birth of your baby to use them.

- **You may develop the "mask of pregnancy."** Pregnancy holds an additional risk of suntanning called melasma (or chloasma), a pigment change on the face commonly referred to as the mask of pregnancy. It is most common in women with darker complexions. While sunblocks are somewhat effective at preventing this, the best approach is to shade your face with a large hat or to stay out of the sun altogether. Once melasma develops, it may last throughout your pregnancy. And although it tends to fade with time, the affected areas may never regain their normal appearance.

- **A faint dark line may form from your navel to your pubic area.** This is known as the linea nigra, and it's a temporary mark caused by pregnancy hormones. It will disappear as the top layers of skin cells are shed a month or two after delivery.

- **You may develop skin tags.** The hormones of pregnancy also contribute to the development of little flaps of skin that appear on your breasts, armpits, or neck. Unfortunately, these so-called skin tags will not miraculously disappear after delivery. However, your doctor can remove them with a simple procedure.

PARENT TO PARENT
*"I got the itchiest legs while I was
pregnant, and I found out that the
greatest thing was lots of high-quality
lotion like Cetaphil. If your bath or shower
water is too hot or you stay in too long, it
can actually make your skin worse in the
long run. After your bath, make sure you
put on the lotion while your skin is still
damp. Shave a little less often, too! I am
now 20 weeks and the itching has
stopped. What a relief!"*

—**momof7sofar,** AS POSTED ON DRSPOCK.COM

Your hair is likely to change

Pregnancy can do many different things to your hair—
some good and some not so good. If you have naturally
curly hair, you may notice that it becomes straighter when
you're pregnant. After you deliver, it will probably go back
to being curly, though not always. Some mothers-to-be
become aware of hair sprouting where they are not used
to seeing it, such as on their ever-growing abdomens.
Many notice that the hair on their heads becomes thicker
during pregnancy. Unfortunately, all good things must

come to an end. A few months after giving birth, much of this newly luxuriant hair tends to fall out. This is normal in the postpartum period. Your hair should return to normal within a few months after delivery.

If you color or perm your hair, you may be wondering if it's safe to continue these treatments while you're pregnant. The answer is: probably. Both processes involve putting chemicals on your hair that are applied directly to your scalp. Small amounts of the chemicals do get into your bloodstream. In animal studies, hair chemicals have been linked to birth defects, but only with much larger exposure than you get with routine hair procedures. While there is no actual evidence that hair dye is harmful during pregnancy, many practitioners recommend not dying hair in the first trimester, when the fetal organs are forming. Processes like highlighting, which don't contact the scalp, are preferable because they don't get into your body.

Another important consideration before you plunk down money on hair treatments is that your hair may not respond the way it usually does. Hairstylists tell me that a perm may leave their pregnant clients' hair straight or exceedingly frizzy, or may even cause a wave in some places and not in others—probably not the look you were going for!

Nails are affected too

While you're pregnant, your nails tend to grow faster than they did before. Many women find that a manicure or pedicure is a way of providing a welcome lift to their spirits. Later in pregnancy, a professional pedicure also may take care of the increasingly difficult task of cutting your toenails, as your belly begins to interfere with your ability to reach your own feet. The fumes from chemicals that sometimes go along with manicures and pedicures, however, can be a source of concern. Try to make sure that you are in a relatively open area, that there is plenty of ventilation in the room, and that you are not exposed to the fumes for a long period of time.

Q: Are massages safe in pregnancy?

A: Many pregnant women find that a massage is an excellent way to rejuvenate and relax. If it is uncomfortable for you to lie on your tummy, try lying on your side, or sitting backward on a straight-backed chair for a back massage. Many massage therapists offer a table made especially for pregnant women with a cutout in the middle for your pregnant belly. Massaging the abdomen can lead to contractions. If you notice this, it is probably best not to continue this part of the massage. Keep in mind that you are doing this to help yourself relax. Don't do anything that doesn't feel good.

GETTING GOOD CARE

While many prenatal visits focus on both you and your baby, the fourth-month visit is often all about the baby.

The mother-to-be is generally feeling pretty well, and this is the most stable time of pregnancy in terms of complications. Your practitioner will measure the size of your uterus and compare it with how many weeks along you are supposed to be; this is the visit where twins may be suspected if your uterus suddenly seems too big. During your fourth month, if not earlier, your practitioner will offer testing for genetic problems. Depending on your age, you may be encouraged to undergo amniocentesis or to have a blood test called a triple (or quadruple) check.

Amniocentesis offers a check of fetal chromosomes

In amniocentesis, using ultrasound to guide the procedure, your doctor will insert a long needle through your abdomen to remove a sample of amniotic fluid from the sac that surrounds your baby. This probably sounds pretty painful, but it really hurts only about as much as a regular shot. And like a shot, it's for a good cause: Amniocentesis can uncover many congenital conditions, alerting you to potential problems (or, even better, providing some peace of mind about your baby's health). Amniocentesis is usually performed at around 16 weeks' gestation, although sometimes it can be done earlier in pregnancy.

Once the fluid has been collected, your doctor will send it off to a medical lab for an analysis of the chromosome content of the fetal cells. In Down syndrome and some other conditions, for example, there are an abnormal number of chromosomes in each cell, which the tests are very accurate about detecting. There are now also many tests for more subtle genetic conditions. Genetic counseling before amniocentesis can determine which tests should be done on a case-by-case basis.

In addition, amniocentesis fluid also can be analyzed for alpha-fetoprotein (AFP). High levels of AFP are a sign of possible body-cavity malformations such as spina bifida, in which the spinal membranes or cord can protrude from the fetus's spinal column, resulting in paralysis or other serious problems. While blood levels of AFP are part of the routine triple check test (see page 97), checking the AFP in the amniotic fluid is even more accurate.

When done in the second trimester, amniocentesis involves a slight risk of miscarriage. Ask your practitioner what the specific risk is in the ultrasound unit that will perform your procedure. Usually that risk is about 1 in 200, meaning that 99.5 percent of amniocentesis tests do not cause fetal loss.

Who should have amniocentesis?
The risk of Down syndrome slowly increases with the mother's age. At 35 years of age, women have a risk of about 1 in 200 of giving birth to a baby with Down syndrome. By age 40, the risk is about 1 in 100, and at 45, it jumps to 1 in 50. The risk level might be calculated by the mother's age alone, or in combination with her triple check results (see page 97). In the United States, standard care is to offer amniocentesis to all women who have more than a 1-in-200 chance of identifying a genetic problem in the fetus.

Of course, this offer represents a value judgment that does not hold in all families. For some, any risk of Down syndrome feels unacceptable, and a young woman may choose to have amniocentesis even though the risk of the test's causing a miscarriage is higher than the chance of Down syndrome in her case. For others, the possibility of causing the loss of an otherwise healthy pregnancy feels unacceptable, and they choose to decline amniocentesis, even if they are at high risk of finding a problem. This is often the case with older moms who have gone through infertility treatment and

PARENT TO PARENT

"I ended up having an amnio last Tuesday. It's been four days and I am fine. It's not a fun thing to do—just like a shot, it stings at first and you feel some pressure, but mainly it's just scary. Afterward, they made me rest at home for two days—no working, riding in the car, nothing but sitting on my butt! That gives the tiny pierced hole time to completely close up. I only experienced slight cramping and soreness. I'm glad I did it, because the amnio came back negative for birth defects, so I can finish out the rest of my pregnancy with fewer worries."

—**MommyCoogs,** AS POSTED ON DRSPOCK.COM

who feel they cannot risk losing the pregnancy under any circumstances. In still other cases, the parents know that they wouldn't terminate a pregnancy for Down syndrome and don't see any reason to do the testing.

Triple check and other tests provide alternatives

Research is currently under way to find a method to extract fetal cells from the mother's blood. If this procedure becomes viable, under many circumstances a simple no-risk blood test could be substituted for amniocentesis.

Even before this welcome day arrives, other tests are available to assess fetal chromosomes besides amniocentesis. Chorionic villi sampling (CVS) can be done earlier than amniocentesis (around 10 to 11 weeks' gestation) but may carry a slightly higher risk of causing a miscarriage. It is particularly useful in situations where there is a high likelihood of finding a genetic problem, such as in couples who both carry a serious recessive genetic trait, giving their baby a 25 percent chance of being affected. If you think that CVS may make sense in your case, be sure to discuss this alternative to amniocentesis with your practitioner or genetics counselor early in your pregnancy.

The triple check test, sometimes called the triple screen, is an optional blood test that can indicate an increased risk of spina bifida or Down syndrome as well as some other serious congenital problems. The current standard is a series of three tests that are obtained from the mother's blood, measuring hCG (a pregnancy hormone), estriol (an estrogen made by the placenta), and alpha-fetoprotein (AFP, a protein in the blood of the fetus)—hence the name *triple check*. The results of these three tests, plus the mother's age and weight and the gestational age of the fetus, are then fed into a computer, and out pops an assessment of the risks for that pregnancy. Accurate standards for the triple check test results are not available until about 16 weeks' gestation. Other combinations of blood tests are being developed to improve the accuracy of this screen and to allow testing earlier in pregnancy. Your practitioner can tell you which tests are recommended in your specific situation.

For the risk of Down syndrome, the results are reported as a ratio. A 1-in-5,000 risk of Down syndrome would be a very low risk, and would not require further testing; a 1-in-10 risk would be considered high, and amniocentesis would be recommended. Even with a high risk level like 1:10, though, the chances are good (in this case, 90 percent) that the baby will *not* have Down syndrome. An abnormal result on the triple check test only means that more testing is indicated.

For the risk of spina bifida and other open-body-cavity problems, the results are reported as "normal" (no further testing recommended) or "increased" (further testing is recommended). Usually the test is repeated, and if the second triple check is again abnormal, the next step is an in-depth ultrasound, which allows a detailed look at the fetal anatomy. If that result isn't clear, amniocentesis is sometimes recommended.

An abnormal test doesn't automatically mean an unhealthy baby

Remember that most babies with abnormal screening results are actually doing just fine. There is a big overlap between the results from healthy babies and the results of fetuses with problems, which means that a lot of people with perfectly normal babies have a scare when they go through amniocentesis or an in-depth ultrasound. That's very unfortunate, but until the tests are further refined to make them more accurate, it's the only way to be sure that most fetuses with these problems are identified. Also, since the normal values of the triple check are very dependent on how far along you are in pregnancy, sometimes after ultrasound a new due date can be identified and the triple check results can be reanalyzed with this in mind. Many times the triple check is normal when the new due date is taken into account.

There are two general reasons why some people choose not to have the triple check done:

- **They're going to have amniocentesis and ultrasound anyway.** The triple check only helps to identify which moms-to-be should have amnio or ultrasound done. If you are going to have either or both of these procedures anyway, the triple check serves no real purpose. Many (but not all) women who will be 35 years old at delivery fall into this category.

- **They're going to have an in-depth ultrasound but would decline amniocentesis even if it were recommended.** Again, the triple check is to see who needs further testing, and if the testing will be declined no matter what, why do the triple check? Many (but not all) people who would not terminate a Down syndrome pregnancy fall into this category.

It is important to think through what you will do with the information you get from your triple check test. If that information will help you make decisions about your pregnancy, then you probably should get the blood test done. If you are not willing to get the further testing that might be recommended or would carry on your pregnancy no matter what, it may be better to forgo the triple check rather than spend the rest of your pregnancy worrying about any distressing test results.

A NOTE FOR PEOPLE WHO ARE NOT GOING TO HAVE AN ULTRASOUND 🏍

The triple check also can give a hint of findings usually seen on ultrasound: a double-check of the doctor's estimate of the due date, the presence of twins, major and ultimately fatal birth defects such as anencephaly (a rare condition in which part of the skull and most of the brain fail to form), and some anatomical problems that would make vaginal birth unsafe for the baby. If you are not going to have an ultrasound, these other factors should be taken into account when making the decision about triple check.

LOOKING AHEAD

Don't let all this talk about checking for trouble dampen your excitement about pregnancy! As you emerge from the fourth month, and hopefully have found out that all is well, you can begin to really enjoy yourself. Most mothers-to-be spend lots of time wondering what their baby will be like, and how their lives and their relationships will be transformed. If this is your first baby, you may see your interactions with your own parents changing, as well as your relationship with the baby's father. Even your self-image may change as you start to picture yourself as a mom.

Mothers- and fathers-to-be are sometimes concerned about repeating patterns from their pasts. If you think the parenting you received wasn't always healthy, you may worry about your own ability to be a good parent. Even if your parents were wonderful, it can be intimidating to think of yourself in this new role. This is new territory for you. Since you will be very busy after the baby comes, use this time to learn about healthy parenting as well as about pregnancy and birth. Take advantage of resources in the community, such as breastfeeding and infant-care classes, articles and discussions groups on the Web at *www.drSpock.com* and other good parenting sites, and the many books and magazines that are available on these subjects. There is a world of helpful information out there.

Domestic violence and pregnancy

My fondest hope is that you and your baby's father have a wonderful relationship and that you'll be bringing your child into a happy home. But the sad fact is that violence toward a woman by her spouse or partner is very common. Sometimes a woman gets so used to having a threatening or violent partner that she doesn't even realize how bad her situation is. But consider this: Every person has the right to be safe in her home and to be treated with respect by those who claim to care about her. Here is a brief quiz to help you think about your relationship:

1. Do you ever feel unsafe at home?
2. Does your partner frequently belittle, insult, or blame you?
3. Is your partner unreasonably jealous? Has he falsely accused you of infidelity?
4. Has your partner ever threatened you with physical violence?
5. Has your partner ever hit, kicked, slapped, pushed, or choked you?
6. Do you feel controlled or isolated by your partner? Has your freedom been restricted, or are you kept from doing things that are important to you?
7. Does your partner ever try to control you by threatening to hurt your family?
8. Has your partner ever pressured or forced you to perform sexual acts against your will?
9. Many people are more violent when under the influence of drugs or alcohol. Does your partner use drugs

such as "uppers" or amphetamines, speed, angel dust, cocaine, crack, street drugs, heroin, or mixtures? Is he drunk every day or almost every day?

10. Does he threaten to kill you? Whether or not he's issued threats, do you believe he is capable of killing you? Is there a gun in the house?

If the answer to even one question is yes, you should carefully assess your safety in this relationship. Domestic violence often escalates in pregnancy and can result in harm to your developing baby as well as yourself. And after your child is born, there will be two of you to harm. Even if your spouse or partner doesn't directly abuse your child, your baby will still be exposed to very harmful influences: Children who grow up as witnesses of domestic violence tend to become victims or abusers themselves.

I know that it can be very difficult to confront these issues. You may feel financially or emotionally dependent on your partner. But there are ways out. If you have questions or concerns about your safety, talk to your doctor or midwife, get support from friends or family members, or contact a local shelter for abused women. You and your baby deserve a better life!

The second trimester is a good time to travel

Now on to a happier subject. Whether for work, to see family, or to visit someplace new on vacation, travel has become a major part of modern life. The best time for travel in pregnancy is during the second trimester, when most mothers-to-be feel well and pregnancy complications are least likely. In the first trimester, many women feel too fatigued or crummy to go far, especially if they're bothered by vaginal bleeding or significant nausea. Travel also typically isn't recommended late in the third trimester. Many women feel tired and sore, and medical care may be needed if they develop problems or go into labor away from home. If you're considering a third-trimester trip, it's particularly important that you discuss your plans with your practitioner.

Buses, trains, planes, and cars all can be safe, so your mode of travel depends on your own personal preference and your circumstances. Just be sure that your choice allows you to move around during the trip. Do not sit for long periods of time in one position, as sitting still or crossing your legs can cause stiffness and discomfort, not to mention the fact that it adds to your already increased risk of venous thrombosis (blood clots in your legs). To prevent this from happening, get up and walk every two to three hours, do simple leg exercises while sitting (even flexing your feet up and down helps), sit with your legs uncrossed, and try to vary your position as much as possible.

Short-distance travel is generally fine unless you are close to your due date and have reason to expect a short labor. In general, a one-to-two-hour trip poses no specific concerns. Longer domestic trips, of course, take you farther away from your own healthcare professional and chosen birth setting. Generally, this is fine in low-risk pregnancies when childbirth is not imminent. Just be sure to discuss your plans with your practitioner.

International travel is a little more complicated. For travel to modern cities, a copy of your medical record and knowledge of how to contact your embassy may be all that you need. For more exotic locations, requirements for immunizations or antimalarial medications often can be accommodated in pregnancy. But frankly, travel to a developing country or a remote region is risky business when you're pregnant. Think long and hard about the implications of needing emergency medical or obstetrical services in such a setting, and be sure to talk to your practitioner before you commit to such a trip.

BEFORE YOU GO . . . 🏍

Make sure that you're familiar with the results of any tests or ultrasounds you may have had. In many instances, it is sufficient to know that your blood pressure, urine tests, and ultrasound were normal. It is best, however, to actually bring a copy of your medical records with you when you travel, particularly in the third trimester, so that you'll have that information on hand in the event that you require medical care.

Thinking ahead about circumcision

Unless you know for sure that you're going to have a girl, it's a good idea for you and your partner to discuss cir-

CAR TRAVEL ALLOWS THE MOST FLEXIBILITY 🌿

*In some ways, traveling by car is the best way to go
in pregnancy. You have room for your personal
items, and you have control over when you stop and
when you travel. Two important considerations:*

Wear a seat belt. *You might think that a seat belt
would put too much pressure on the baby in the
event of an accident, but that's not the case.
Numerous studies have shown that both mother
and fetus are safest if the mom is buckled in. This is
probably because in order for the fetus to survive,
his mother must survive the accident as well—and
that's much more likely, of course, if she is belted in.
Wear the lap belt low and snug below your tummy,
make sure that the shoulder belt falls across your
shoulder and abdomen, and push your seat as far
back as you can in order to keep as much distance
as possible between you and the airbag.*

Take lots of breaks. *Yes, it can be frustrating to add
time to an already long trip, but it's important to
take frequent breaks from sitting. Otherwise, you'll
increase your risk of developing blood clots because
of pooling of blood in the leg veins combined with
the increased clotting factors in pregnancy. Walking
around for about 10 minutes every two to three
hours keeps your blood circulating.*

cumcision in case your special delivery turns out to be a boy. Circumcision is a minor surgical procedure to remove the foreskin, a flap of skin that covers the tip of the penis.

Circumcision is sometimes done as a religious observance (as in Islam and Judaism). Other parents opt for circumcision for cosmetic reasons, so that a boy will look "like his father," or like the other guys in the locker room (well, American locker rooms, anyway).

In 1999, an expert panel of the American Academy of Pediatrics concluded that circumcision does have some demonstrated medical benefits. For example, circumcised infants are significantly less likely to develop infections of the bladder and kidneys. Circumcision also seems to reduce the risk of developing penile cancer and certain sexually transmitted diseases. However, the expert panel did not feel that these benefits were large enough to justify recommending that all baby boys undergo this small surgical procedure.

Newborn circumcisions are usually done by the obstetrician or family doctor who delivers the baby. Some nurse-midwives also do circumcisions. In some regions it is the pediatricians, instead of the obstetrical practitioners, who perform the procedure. Urologists generally do circumcisions only on older children and adults (in an operating room with general anesthesia), although occasionally they may be called on to circumcise a newborn with unusual anatomy.

Nonritual circumcision usually is done within the

FLYING THE FRIENDLY SKIES 🐞

I have a fantasy about someday being on a flight, hearing a passenger call out for a doctor because a woman has gone into labor, and coming to her rescue. Understandably, the airlines would rather this heroic scenario not come to pass. They don't want to be responsible for complications of pregnancy or childbirth, so if you are visibly pregnant, airline personnel may give you a hard time when you show up for your trip. Whether you are near your due date or just look that way, it's a good idea to bring a note from your practitioner saying that he has deemed it safe for you to travel by air.

Many women wonder if the oxygen levels in the plane cabins are safe for their developing babies. The answer is yes if we're talking about commercial

first few days of birth. It takes between one and five minutes and involves creating a thin ring of crushed tissue at the base of the foreskin where the incision is then made. The crushing of the tissue prevents bleeding. There are different sorts of instruments for protecting the tip of the penis during the procedure. Most practitioners have one technique with which they are most comfortable. Complications of circumcision, such as bleeding and infection, are rare. Very rarely, a major complication can occur due to surgical mishap.

Traditionally, no anesthetic was used for circumcision.

airplanes, which are pressurized at the equivalent of an altitude of 8,000 feet. This provides plenty of oxygen for you and your fetus, although you may notice mild shortness of breath during the flight. Small private planes, however, may not be as well pressurized as commercial airliners, and so are best avoided during pregnancy. And if you have any significant medical problems such as lung or heart disease, you should discuss with your practitioner whether air travel is wise.

Finally, just as with car travel, it's a good idea to stretch your legs often while flying in a plane. Do a few stretching exercises while you're sitting in your seat to keep the blood circulating through your legs, and frequent strolls down the aisle to get your circulation moving. (Your bladder probably won't let you sit for more than a few hours at a time, anyway!)

However, experts now agree that infants do feel pain. In studies that compared using local anesthesia with no anesthetic, for example, the babies cried less, maintained a more normal heart rate during the procedure, and were less irritable afterward when local anesthesia was used.

Many practitioners now use one of three local anesthetic techniques:

• Topical anesthetic (EMLA) cream can be put on about an hour before the procedure to numb the skin. This is the least invasive method of anesthesia, but it isn't as effective as the other two methods.

- Ring block (local anesthesia) is done by injecting a local anesthetic (like the kind the dentist uses) around the base of the foreskin near where the incision will be made.
- Penile block (nerve block) is done by injecting local anesthetic at the base of the penis, where the nerves for pain are located.

Other methods of calming a newborn during circumcision include giving a pacifier, stroking him, and talking quietly to him.

NOTES

Use this space to jot down observations about your pregnancy or questions to ask your healthcare practitioner at your next visit:

_____

_____

_____

_____

_____

_____

_____

_____

_____

_____

_____

_____

_____

CHAPTER 5

Weeks 18–22

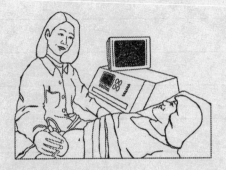

At this point in your pregnancy, your doctor or midwife is likely to recommend that you have an ultrasound examination. This procedure uses harmless ultrasonic waves to produce images of your uterus and fetus. It can help your practitioner assess everything from the accuracy of your due date to how well your baby is growing.

ABOUT YOUR BABY

This month, you will pass the midpoint of your pregnancy. In the first half of gestation, your little embryo has gone from a few cells to a complex being with all her organs in place. She even has fingernails and toenails. She moves her arms and legs, and on ultrasound, you may catch her sucking her thumb.

You may be feeling your baby move every day, or you may not yet notice her flutters and pokes. First-time moms tend to feel their babies' activity later than you might think: around 20 or even 23 weeks. Experienced moms often notice fetal movement as early as 15 weeks. This is probably because once they have felt their babies move in a prior pregnancy, they recognize the sensation earlier the next time around. As babies get bigger and stronger, their movements become unmistakable.

Q: I am in my 21st week of pregnancy. I have felt my baby move often except for the last three days, during which time I have felt only one or two movements. Is this normal or should I be worried?

A: In the second trimester, your awareness of fetal activity can vary from day to day. It is not unusual to feel the baby one day and not feel him much the next. I don't think anyone knows if this is because a baby's movements are truly that variable, or if a mother just fails to notice them sometimes.

I certainly wouldn't worry right now, but in your third trimester it would be unusual to go a whole day without feeling the baby move. If you notice anything like this at that time, be sure to let your doctor or midwife know about your situation.

ABOUT YOU

Babies are nutrition magnets! Drawing upon their mothers' bodies, they help themselves to everything that they need. And as they get bigger, their nutritional needs increase. That's why eating a healthy, well-balanced diet isn't so much to ensure that your baby gets what he needs but so that *you* have enough left for yourself. If you have bad eating habits or are on a restricted diet, if you know you are deficient in a specific nutrient, or if you are overweight, underweight, or have an eating disorder, a consultation with a nutritionist can help you and your baby stay healthy.

Supplements help ensure adequate nutrition

After the embryonic organs have formed in the early first trimester, taking folate (see page 4) is no longer so crucial. If you're a healthy woman who eats a balanced diet, it is reasonable to think of routine prenatal vitamins as an insurance policy against the unlikely chance that you are not getting enough of one of the many nutrients recommended for pregnancy. But for many women, even a good diet and prenatal vitamins may not supply all the calcium and iron they need as their pregnancy progresses.

Iron is essential to red blood cells

Iron is important to build the baby's blood cells, as well as to maintain yours. How much iron you need during pregnancy depends both on how much you already have stored in your bone marrow and how much you get in your diet. For meat-eaters, the amount in any multivitamin labeled "with iron" will probably be enough, at least in the first half of pregnancy. Most practitioners will check your blood count (or hemoglobin level) early in your pregnancy, and then again around the seventh month, prescribing extra iron if needed. Some routinely recommend extra iron tablets to all their patients throughout pregnancy, especially for those with risk factors for deficiency in this mineral, such as poor nutrition or closely spaced pregnancies.

Babies are very good at getting all the iron they need from their mothers' storehouses of the mineral. They take more toward the end of pregnancy, as they get bigger and produce more red blood cells. It is rare for a newborn to have iron-deficiency anemia (low red blood cells), even if the mother is low on iron herself.

Mothers, on the other hand, often end up slightly anemic by the end of pregnancy. There is some evidence that severe anemia in a pregnant woman is associated with low-birth-weight babies and preterm birth. It isn't clear if this is cause and effect, or if women who are very anemic have other problems, like poverty, that put them at greater risk.

If a woman has a low red blood cell count when she goes into labor, she may get to a dangerously low level if she bleeds more than usual during childbirth. While it is rare for a mother to need a blood transfusion around the time of delivery, it makes sense that the higher the blood count in late pregnancy, the larger the safety net.

The most common iron-related problem in pregnancy is that taking two or more iron supplements a day can cause abdominal cramping, dark green and grainy stools, and constipation. Even the small amount of iron in a prenatal vitamin can cause some women to become constipated; conversely, some people get diarrhea from iron. Depending on how much you need this mineral, you may be able to decrease your iron intake, or you may have to treat the intestinal symptoms so that you can continue the iron.

Pickles and ice cream, anyone?

Along with all the healthy foods and supplements moms-to-be are diligent about consuming, many report strong food cravings during their pregnancies. Sometimes it's an overwhelming urge to indulge in a certain favorite food on a daily basis. Sometimes it's a sudden desire for a food they normally dislike, or for a weird combination of foods. And occasionally it's not for a food at all: Pregnant moms have been known to develop a taste for clay, dirt, or other substances not normally found on the family dinner table; these abnormal cravings are known as pica (pronounced PIE-ka). A sampling of the unusual dietary urges moms-to-be have posted on the drSpock.com message boards appears on pages 118–19.

Calcium is the key to building healthy bones

Calcium is important in building your baby's bones as well as maintaining your own bone density. While prenatal vitamins have some calcium, none have enough to satisfy the prenatal requirement; the pill would have to be the size of a robin's egg! Usually 1,500 mg of calcium per day is recommended for pregnant women, the equivalent of five helpings of milk, cheese, yogurt, or ice cream. Calcium

SOME IRONCLAD INFORMATION 🏍

- Red meat (including liver and kidney), poultry, and fish are good sources of digestible iron.

- The iron in fruits and vegetables is absorbed best if you take vitamin C or eat a little meat at the same time.

- Coffee and tea (even the decaffeinated varieties), foods high in dietary fiber (such as bran), calcium supplements, and antacids consumed within two hours of eating iron-rich foods can decrease iron absorption.

- Many cereals and breads are fortified with extra iron. Check the labels.

- Ferrous sulfate is the most common over-the-counter iron supplement, but it can cause stomach upset or constipation. Ferro-sequels are ferrous sulfate with a stool softener right in the pill. Ferrous gluconate, especially in the liquid form, may be the easiest on the GI tract and is at least as effective as ferrous sulfate.

- Take only the dose recommended by your practitioner. The body cannot absorb more than about two standard iron supplements a day, so taking more is not helpful—and very hard on the digestive tract. Besides, over time, taking too much iron can be toxic to the liver and other vital organs. (Note: If you have a young child at home, be sure to keep your iron supplements or multivitamins containing iron in childproof containers and out of his reach.)

PARENT TO PARENT

"I'm craving salt-and-vinegar chips with peanut butter (in fact, that sounds good right now!), along with pickles with cashews and raspberries. I'm eating so much of these things, it's unbelievable."

—PamExpectinTwins

"With my first baby, I craved salt like crazy and always wanted McDonald's cheeseburgers—something I never ate before and haven't eaten since. Oh, and lots of green olives."

—momof7sofar

"The weirdest craving I got was apples and tomato sauce. When I think of that now, I just say, 'EWWWWWWWW!' "

—3California_Kids

intake becomes more important as the pregnancy progresses and the baby's need for this element increases.

Be particularly careful to get enough calcium in the second half of pregnancy, as the baby gets bigger and is taking more from you. Most women in the United States don't get enough calcium in their diets, even

"Chocolate ice cream with potato chips is
my strangest craving this time. My first
pregnancy was nonstop cravings for
tomatoes with sugar. I HATE TOMATOES
and I always have, but I craved them for
some reason!"

—SanDiegoMoma4

"I don't have any food cravings with my
latest pregnancy, but I have to admit,
for some strange reason, I get this urge
to put talcum powder in a bowl and run
my hands through it. In fact, I would love
to fill up my tub with powder
and get in it."

—mrs.jewelmaker

when they're not pregnant. This is part of the reason
that older women have such a high incidence of hip
fractures. A woman is most able to build bone
strength from her teen years through her thirties. Peak
bone mass is reached by age 35 or even earlier. From
then on, the best you can do with diet and exercise is

maintain your bones—they will not get stronger. In addition to the teen years, after menopause, and during breastfeeding, pregnancy is one of the times in your life when you really need to pay attention to calcium intake. Protect your bones. They must last you a lifetime.

Calcium supplements such as calcium carbonate come in chewable form (like TUMS antacids or VIACTIV soft chews) or as regular pills. Some include vitamin D or other vitamins or minerals. In pregnancy, plain old calcium carbonate is fine. The biggest problem with any of the calcium supplements is constipation. Pregnancy can be constipating enough without adding this insult. If you are struggling with this problem, try to get calcium from your food rather than supplements, or try some of the preventive measures for constipation in pregnancy (see page 196).

If you are going to take supplements, one option is to take five or more TUMS, spaced out during the day. This method is a favorite of heartburn sufferers. Another method is to take one 500 or 600 mg calcium pill in the morning, and then take another in the evening if you haven't gotten a lot of dietary calcium that day. This can increase your awareness of your diet and, with any luck, gets you enough calcium without taking more pills than your GI tract can handle.

Heartburn plagues many mothers-to-be

Most women experience burning in the middle of the chest, belching, or the taste of acid in the throat

GOOD DIETARY SOURCES OF CALCIUM 🌾

Each of the following has about 300 mg of calcium, a fifth of what a pregnant woman usually needs each day:

- One glass of milk
- One cup of calcium-fortified juice
- One TUMS EX or 1½ regular TUMS
- A 4-ounce tin of canned sardines or salmon
- A 12-ounce milkshake
- One serving of lasagna
- 1½ cups of ice cream (along with a lot of calories!)
- One cup of yogurt
- A 2-ounce serving of American cheese
- Just over a cup of cooked spinach
- One cup of Total cereal

Note: While broccoli has the reputation for providing calcium, one 8-ounce serving has only about 100 milligrams.

at some point in pregnancy—and often at many points. Heartburn and indigestion are part and parcel of normal pregnancy. You may already be taking calcium-based antacids, such as TUMS, as an extra source of calcium, and if they help your heartburn, too, that's great. However, calcium-based antacids usually aren't sufficient for severe or persistent heartburn.

Heartburn is caused by stomach acid passing up into the esophagus (food tube), a process called reflux. The pregnancy hormone progesterone slows digestion and causes delay in the stomach emptying after meals. At the same time, it allows the sphincter muscle at the top of the stomach to relax. With the stomach full of food and acid, and the valve at the top not staying shut, it can be a real double whammy, allowing acid to go up and burn the esophagus. Lying down when the stomach is full makes reflux even worse.

PARENT TO PARENT
"Well, they say that the more heartburn you have when you're pregnant, the more hair the baby has. I had horrible heartburn with my son and he had a LOT of hair, so maybe it's true! With that pregnancy, nothing seemed to help, but with this one, my doctor tells me to take TUMS and Maalox and avoid food that gives me heartburn. Easier said than done, because everything seems to!"

—**MaMi4ThE2ndTiMe,** AS POSTED ON DRSPOCK.COM

What can you do about heartburn?

- **Diet.** Eat small amounts of food at a time so the stomach has less to empty. Avoid peppermints, caffeine, and alcohol, which stimulate acid production and further relax the sphincter. Try to finish dinner early in the evening, and don't lie down after eating.

- **Activities.** Sleep propped up in a semisitting position, or raise the head of your bed by putting two of its legs up on cinder blocks.

- **Medications.** Women who don't have major medical problems can safely take antacids in pregnancy.

  ○ Calcium-based antacids aren't the most effective; while they provide a great source of calcium and temporarily neutralize acid, they cause your stomach to increase its production of acid an hour after they are taken.

  ○ Mylanta, Maalox, and other magnesium-based antacids seem to give longer-lasting relief of symptoms. Many women find that the liquid form works best, even though chewables are most convenient. In healthy women, the dosage of these medications is not critical. It is fine to keep a bottle by the bed and take a gulp or two during the night when necessary. If you get diarrhea—which is the most common side effect of magnesium-based antacids—you will need to decrease the amount you are taking or try a different treatment.

  ○ Over-the-counter stomach-acid blockers (such as Pepcid, Tagamet, and Zantac) are probably safe in pregnancy. Do not exceed the recommended dose without checking with your doctor.

o Prescription medications are also available. Sucral-fate liquid (Carafate) is an excellent choice since it is not absorbed into the body. It simply coats the stomach and esophagus. Its one drawback is that it can be constipating. Ask your doctor or nurse-midwife if it would be a good choice for you.

Acid reflux and indigestion are not dangerous, just annoying and sometimes very uncomfortable side effects of being pregnant. Luckily, most women get good relief with proper treatment. If your symptoms don't respond to a change in your habits or over-the-counter therapies, talk to your practitioner about what else can be done.

Pregnancy makes you more prone to excessive bleeding

Many expectant mothers find that they get occasional nosebleeds while they're pregnant. The nosebleeds are caused by swelling and increased blood supply to the nasal passages. They usually can be treated with pres-sure on the bridge of the nose or an ice pack, just like nosebleeds at other times.

You also may notice that your gums bleed when you brush or floss your teeth. The culprit usually is gingivitis (from *gingiva*, meaning gums, and *-itis*, meaning inflammation). Food particles that get caught between the teeth and gums attract bacteria, which can lead to inflammation. This condition can plague anyone, but the hormones of pregnancy often aggravate it by causing tissues to swell and increasing the supply of blood to the gums.

The best way to keep gingivitis at bay is to brush and floss regularly. Foods with hard slivers, like popcorn, have a particular tendency to stick between the teeth and gums and should be flossed out as soon as possible or, better yet, avoided. Contact your dentist if your gums continue to bleed several minutes after brushing. There is some evidence that gum disease is connected with poor pregnancy outcomes, including premature birth. It may just be that people with severe gum disease aren't taking good care of themselves in general, but it is worthwhile to take your dental care seriously, especially during pregnancy. Be sure to tell your dentist that you are pregnant, and remember that you shouldn't have X rays or take medication unless it's absolutely necessary.

Occasionally, pregnant women experience a problem with the blood's ability to clot. If, in addition to bleeding gums, you bruise easily, have frequent or heavy nosebleeds, or experience bleeding in other parts of your body, let your practitioner know.

GETTING GOOD CARE

In the fifth month, the prenatal visit usually includes routine checks of your blood pressure and weight, urine testing for sugar and protein, and a "tummy check." Your uterus has expanded to the level of your belly button at 20 weeks, give or take a couple of inches. This visit is usually medically uncomplicated, and can be a good time to bring up any questions you have as you start planning for labor and birth.

Listening to the heartbeat without amplification

While your practitioner will probably listen to the baby with the amplified Doppler instrument, the heartbeat actually can be heard without electronic amplification starting at about 20 weeks. A special stethoscope called a fetoscope can be used, or the bell (concave) side of a regular stethoscope can be pressed firmly onto your abdomen. The heartbeat is best heard over the baby's back, which often feels like a fairly broad, firm area when you press around on your uterus. If you are overweight or if the placenta is on the front wall of the uterus, it may be difficult to hear the fetal heart with a stethoscope. It gets easier later in the pregnancy.

Ultrasound provides a window into your baby's world

Your doctor or midwife may recommend getting an ultrasound to confirm your due date and check the fetal anatomy. While there isn't any research that has shown that babies do better with routine ultrasound, many practitioners (and parents) still feel most comfortable if they have "seen" the fetus before birth. Ultrasound is believed to be safe, but there is a financial cost—around $200 to $400—that may cause some insurance companies to balk at paying for it on a routine basis (that is, not for a specific medical reason).

Depending on such technical factors as fetal position, ultrasound can provide images of the baby that help us assess his welfare. By 18 weeks' gestation, ultrasound often can see external features such as the baby's head, chest, abdomen, genitalia, arms, legs, hands, and feet, as well as some internal features such as the bladder, spine, heart, liver, stomach, and kidneys. In addition, ultrasound can help assess:

- the position of the baby
- how well he's growing
- if the amniotic-fluid volume is high, low, or average
- the location of the placenta
- if the mother's cervix is starting to change
- the presence of fibroids (usually benign tumors) on the mother's uterus.

What ultrasound cannot do

Ultrasound looks at the physical characteristics of your baby. When a clear view is obtained, the sonographer often can be certain of details such as how many chambers are in the heart or that the spine is intact. But sometimes there is uncertainty: Maybe the normal structure was not seen well, or something out of the ordinary was present. This may require a consultation with a specialist or a repeat ultrasound later in the pregnancy, when the organs are larger. And keep in mind that, while it's a highly useful tool, ultrasound can miss important findings. It sometimes can pick up a hint of a congenital abnormality, but it cannot identify

PARENT TO PARENT

"I know that a lot of people are crazed to know if they're having a boy or girl when they go in for an ultrasound. I was curious, too, but when I saw that fuzzy, black-and-white image on the screen—moving, no less!—I forgot all about the boy-girl stuff. I was just amazed and humbled by this first glimpse of my baby. It made him or her real."

—**StillLearning,** AS POSTED ON DRSPOCK.COM

___

all babies with problems. Nonstructural problems, such as autism, cerebral palsy, chemical abnormalities, and mental retardation, cannot be detected by ultrasound.

Determining due date with ultrasound

Early in the pregnancy, a measurement called crown-rump length is used to determine gestational age. Later, the leg-bone (or femur) length and a measurement across the head (biparietal diameter, or BPD) are used. You might be surprised to learn that measurements of the fetus are most precise in determining gestational age in the first trimester (accurate to within one week), less exact in the second trimester (within two weeks), and least accurate in the third

Q: I just had my first ultrasound and the technician told us that, since he couldn't see any evidence of a penis or testicles, we were having a girl. My husband and I are so excited! But we're also a little worried that the ultrasound guy could be wrong. How sure can we be about the sex of our baby?

A: If you are willing to tolerate a small chance that you are telling everyone the wrong sex, go ahead and start announcing and shopping, but you may find yourself returning a lot of pink and frilly things to the stores. It's true that today's refined ultrasound equipment often can identify female genitals with good accuracy. However, even the most experienced ultrasound technician or doctor can't always tell the sex if the baby isn't positioned just right, with a clear view of the genital area. If a tech or doctor doesn't see evidence of male genitals, sometimes he'll tell the parents that it looks as if they're having a girl. But I have seen many a "girl" surprise his parents at birth. Make sure that the tech actually has observed the labia, which look like three parallel lines, before turning to the female section in the baby-names book!

trimester as the baby gets larger (they can be off by three weeks). That's because by the third trimester, different babies grow at very different rates, with some destined to be five-pounders and some to be pushing the ten-pound mark at birth, so size becomes a much less precise gauge of fetal age. If more than one ultrasound is done during pregnancy, the earliest one is the most accurate and will be used to confirm the due date.

LOOKING AHEAD

While labor is but one day in your life, the product of that labor—your baby—will be around for a long time. The name that you choose for her will become part of every day of your life—and hers. You may already have a name picked out. I know couples who picked out names for girls and boys when they were in the early stages of dating, long before they could have known that they would really be having a family together! But for most of us, the decision about names becomes a recurring topic of conversation during pregnancy.

How do you make such a momentous decision? You may want to start by thinking about whether you want the baby named after someone specific, or if you want to choose a name by its sound or meaning. Baby-name books can be a great source of ideas. Do you want a common name or one that is off the beaten path? And will it be OK with you if teachers and others have difficulty with its pronunciation or spelling? Do you like the nicknames that go with a particular name? Many couples make lists of names that they like, and then see which names are on both parents' lists. You can also each eliminate from the other partner's list names that you find unacceptable as you continue to narrow it down. At the end of these steps, there should be some names that you can both agree on. If not, sometimes parents resort to one's picking the name for the first child, while the other gets to pick the next child's moniker.

One word to the wise: If you don't want friends and family members to weigh in on your decision (boy, do people have strong opinions about this topic!), consider announcing the name only *after* the baby is born. At that point, the decision has been made, and there won't be as much of a tendency for everyone to try to sway your choice.

PARENT TO PARENT

"My advice to parents who are agonizing about a name for their baby is this: Just remember that whatever name you pick, it doesn't matter what it sounds like now. Once your baby is born and you started calling him or her that name, it will sound perfect."

—**JodisMom,** AS POSTED ON DRSPOCK.COM

WHAT'S IN A NAME? 🐎

Names influence the children and adults who bear them. Research into the psychology of names has shown that children with less desirable names tend to have lower self-esteem, get poorer grades, and have more psychological problems than those endowed with more popular ones. Adults with unusual names may have a harder time getting elected to public office. But before you decide that John and Ann are the only way to go, remember that there are people with uncommon names who are remarkably successful (ever heard of a man named Keanu or a woman named Oprah?). Besides, many people who grow up with unusual names revel in their uniqueness, while those who are given common names may chafe at being so "ordinary."

With all that's riding on a name, no wonder that parents-to-be spend endless hours mulling—and sometimes fighting—over what to call their babies. Parents choose names for many different reasons: to honor a relative or a famous person they admire, to carry on their own name (think of all the Jr.'s and III's out there), to implant a desired quality (for example, Chastity), or just because the name sounds good.

Cord-blood banking may prove to be a lifesaver later on

Not nearly as much fun to contemplate as names, the issue of whether or not to store some of your baby's

*Perhaps one reason parents spend so much
energy deciding on a name is that a child's
physique, temperament, and talents are
fundamentally out of their control. The name is
one thing that they can actually determine. Often
they try to peer into the future and come up with
names that fit their children, and it truly is
remarkable how often a person's name seems to
suit his personality. By the same token, it can be
quite noticeable when the fit is bad (imagine a
"Tiger" who is meek and studious).*

*In the end, no matter how hard they try, parents
can't be certain how the name they settle on will
affect their child. Perhaps what's important is not so
much picking the "perfect" name, but rather helping
a child grow up strong and confident, able to deal
with both foreseen and unforeseen consequences of
whatever name they choose. (Besides, he can always
resort to a nickname.)*

The article above was written by Dr. Robert
Needlman, a behavioral-developmental
pediatrician who is my colleague at The Dr. Spock
Company.

umbilical-cord blood is something else to consider
well in advance of giving birth. Usually the umbilical
cord—along with the blood that remains in it after a
baby is born and the cord cut—is simply discarded by

the hospital. But in the late 1980s, researchers discovered that cord blood possesses unusual properties
that make it useful in the treatment of patients with
some cancers and other illnesses. It is full of immature cells called stem cells. Unlike *embryonic* stem
cells, which have the ability to develop into any type
of body cell, *cord-blood* stem cells already are locked
into one vital function: making all the different
components of the blood, such as platelets, white
blood cells, and red blood cells—in effect, acting like
bone marrow. When transfused into a patient whose
own blood cells have faulty genetic coding or have
been destroyed by chemotherapy or other cancer
treatments, the cord-blood cells can implant themselves in the bone marrow and generate legions of
new, healthy cells.

These days, umbilical cord-blood transplants are
most commonly used in cancer patients when a donor
can't be found for a bone-marrow transplant. The treatment is particularly effective in young patients. The
University of Colorado Cord Blood Bank reports a 70
percent success rate in children, but only 20 to 40 percent in adults. Researchers envision improving those
odds and see many future applications as well, such as
curing sickle cell disease and other blood-related
genetic illnesses. So there is a possibility that your
child, or someone else, may need these super-healthy
and versatile cells one day.

However, many questions remain. In cancer treatment, for example, some researchers are concerned
about the wisdom of transplanting back into the child

the same cells that already showed a propensity to become malignant. Doctors also aren't sure if the number of cells taken at the time of birth would be enough to treat the child when he is fully grown. It is also not completely clear how active the cells would be after years of being stored. The treatment is so new and rare, we just don't have the experience yet to resolve these important issues.

Aside from these medical uncertainties, the main reason most people do not save their baby's stem cells is cost. In a private cord-blood bank, the initial costs run from $275 to $1,500. Most also charge a yearly storage fee of $50 to $95. When you have a new baby, there are a lot of things to spend that money on. But the advantage of saving cord blood in a private bank is that your sample is saved for only you to use.

Public cord-blood banks are an alternative to saving the blood just for your family. These cost no money, but your sample is not specifically saved for you. Another person with a more immediate need may use it. If the time should come that a member of your family needs stem cells, your baby's may still be available, or you may use donations from others without charge. You also can direct your sample to go to a relative with an immediate need if it matches. Anyone else needing to use stem cells from a public bank who has not been a donor must pay for it—sometimes tens of thousands of dollars.

Each family must weigh the pros and cons for themselves. Some families say that any cost is worth their peace of mind. Others say that in the face of uncertainty about the effectiveness of the treatment, they will use their resources elsewhere. Some choose the no-cost middle ground of donating publicly, knowing that their sample might benefit another family if not themselves. For more information, ask your doctor or nurse, or contact a public or private cord-blood bank.

If you are going to save cord blood, you need to make arrangements with a private or public cord-blood bank, as well as your doctor or midwife, ahead of time. The collection procedure itself is quite simple: After delivery of the baby, the umbilical cord is clamped and cut in the usual way. The blood that remains in the umbilical-cord vessels is then collected in sterile containers. It does not cause the mother or the baby any pain to collect the blood, and no blood is taken that the baby needs at the moment. The nurse, midwife, or physician will then label the samples and package them for a special pickup arranged with a commercial carrier. When the blood arrives at the cord-blood bank, it is processed and the parents are notified. It is then kept in an advanced storage system for years.

NOTES

Use this space to jot down observations about your pregnancy or questions to ask your healthcare practitioner at your next visit:

_____

_____

_____

_____

_____

_____

_____

_____

_____

_____

_____

Weeks 23—26

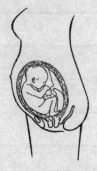

At around 25 weeks, your baby weighs around 1½ pounds and is about a foot long. You're probably feeling him move quite a bit, and he may be in the breech position, as shown here. Don't worry, though: There's still plenty of time for him to drop into the headfirst position that's optimum for birth, as nearly all babies do.

ABOUT YOUR BABY

You are now at the end of the second trimester, and you are probably more and more aware of your baby as a distinct individual, not just an extension of your own body. He is moving around inside your womb every day, and you may often find yourself at odds with each other's moods: When you are trying to rest or pay attention at a meeting, that's likely to be the time your baby decides to practice his kickboxing moves; when you're swimming a few laps or taking a vigorous hike, you may notice that Junior always seems to be napping.

Before 23 to 24 weeks, fetal lungs aren't developed enough to breathe air, a necessary function once a baby is outside the womb and no longer attached to the umbilical cord. Once your baby reaches 23 weeks or so, he still gets his oxygen through the umbilical cord, but he also "breathes" fluid into his lungs, which helps them expand. He's also starting to swallow amniotic fluid into his stomach, which gives his immature digestive system a little practice before milk is introduced after birth.

By the middle of this month (about 25 weeks), your child is likely to weigh about a pound and a half and is roughly 12 inches long. These days, babies born beyond 24 weeks' gestation have a good chance of survival. But your child is still much better off getting his warmth, oxygen, and nutrition through you until after the eighth month of gestation. If born before this time, your baby is likely to be in a neonatal intensive care unit for a while. He may require intravenous feeding, help with breathing, and other high-tech medical care.

ABOUT YOU

At this point in your pregnancy, you may be feeling strong and well, or strained by the physical demands on your body (probably a little of both). One of the less pleasant legacies of pregnancy is stretch marks or striae, the red, pink, or brown lines that you might begin noticing on your abdomen, breasts, or hips. Whether or not you get them is truly a matter of luck (and good genes); some women are riddled with them as their skin stretches to accommodate their growing babies, while others look as fresh and unblemished as Demi Moore on that famous cover of *Vanity Fair.*

Although vitamin E and other treatments have been credited by their manufacturers with preventing striae, none to date have been proven effective. A soothing emollient such as cocoa butter or Aquaphor ointment, though, will help with the itching and dryness that usually accompanies stretch marks.

The good news is that although stretch marks are often bright red and noticeable during pregnancy, they usually slowly change to pink and then grow silvery and pale as time passes. (There is some evidence that applying Retin-A postpartum, while the marks are still red, hastens the fading.) Stretch marks are not usually visible after a few years, and sometimes disappear even sooner. So don't spend your money on ineffective treatments, and try to remember that your skin is stretching for a worthy cause: providing a home for your growing baby.

Sorting out normal abdominal symptoms from preterm labor

Around this time in your pregnancy, you may begin to experience some unusual sensations in your abdomen. Most of the time, these are just normal and benign physical responses, but it can be hard to sort them out from the worrisome symptoms of preterm labor (see page 240). Here's some help in telling the difference:

- **Contractions.** You may notice that your tummy or uterus gets tight or balls up sometimes. These painless, intermittent contractions are a normal part of pregnancy, and are sometimes referred to as Braxton-Hicks contractions. If you tend to have a lot of contractions, it may be difficult to decide if this is premature labor or just a false alarm. If you are less than 35 weeks' pregnant and you have regular contractions lasting more than 30 seconds and occurring more than four to six times an hour, try resting and drinking lots of fluids. If the contractions don't settle down within an hour or two, call your practitioner.

- **Lower back pain.** Pain in the lower back is a common companion in pregnancy. Since some women feel their contractions in their backs, it is important to distinguish normal (if miserable) lower-back pain from contraction pain. If the back pain comes and goes, and your uterus or abdomen is getting tight or hard with the pain, consider the possibility that this pain is from contractions and call your doctor.

- **Blood or mucus from the vagina.** The mucus plug is a jellylike mass that blocks the opening of the cervix. As the cervix starts to get ready for childbirth, the mucus plug may be expelled. This can look like a green glob or like mucus mixed with blood, and often is referred to as the "bloody show." If this happens before 34 weeks, or if you have any bleeding after the first trimester, you should call your practitioner, even if it is after regular office hours.

- **Menstrual-like cramps.** The feeling of menstrual cramps often signifies contractions, even if they are not especially painful. Put your hand on your tummy and see if the uterus is getting hard. If it is, call your doctor or midwife and let her know what's going on.

- **Pelvic or vaginal pressure.** While some pressure is fairly common, especially in mothers who have given birth before, it can be a sign that the cervix is changing without contractions. Severe vaginal or pelvic pressure, particularly if it doesn't resolve with rest, should be reported to your practitioner.

- **Vaginal discharge.** Many women notice an increase in vaginal discharge when they become pregnant. A thin, sticky, clear or white, mild-smelling discharge is usually normal. The amount of discharge generally increases as the pregnancy progresses. To feel fresher, you may find it helpful to wear a panty liner or thin sanitary pad to protect your underwear, and change it frequently. (If your discharge is bloody, watery, changes color, or has a bad odor, or if you are experiencing itching or irritation in your vaginal area, let your practitioner know. This could be a sign of a vaginal infection.)

This discharge is an entirely different situation from the breaking of your bag of waters (see page

238). When your water breaks, you may notice a popping sensation and either a gush or a trickle as some of the amniotic fluid leaks out through your vagina (it may even run down your legs). Some women first notice that their panties are wet. This may continue even after several changes of underwear. In this case, you'll want to put on a sanitary pad and lie down for 30 minutes or so. If you feel a small gush when you get up, it's possible that your amniotic sac has indeed ruptured, and you should call your practitioner to find out what to do next.

Preterm labor involves more than contractions

Preterm labor, also known as premature labor, is the onset of true labor before the 37th week of gestation (three weeks before the due date). In true labor, regular contractions are accompanied by cervical dilation (opening) and effacement (shortening). If there is a change to the cervix without any contractions, or if there are contractions without any cervical change, the condition is not called preterm labor, but it still may affect your care.

Most pregnant women can tell if they are contracting but still require an internal exam to evaluate the cervix. Although the diagnosis usually can be made with physical examination, some other tests may be helpful, including ultrasound to measure the length of the cervix, and a fetal fibronectin test, in which a swab is used to take a cell sample near the cervix. The sample is then sent for analysis at a laboratory. If the fetal fibronectin test comes back negative, it is very unlikely that the woman will deliver in the next two weeks. Even if it comes back positive, it is still more likely that the delivery won't take place, but the healthcare team will watch the mother-to-be more closely and may treat her with medications to stop contractions.

Some preterm labors just stop on their own for no apparent reason. Conversely, some cannot be stopped, even with the use of medication. In many cases, the labor is stopped, but only temporarily. If preterm labor starts but then is stopped and the baby is delivered at term, the baby is at no increased risk for complications. If the labor results in premature delivery, however, the ensuing complications depend on the baby's age, weight, and general condition. The best way to minimize risks from preterm labor is to consult with your practitioner promptly if you are having any worrisome symptoms.

Who is at risk for premature labor?

The majority of women who deliver early don't have any particular risk factors that might warn of an impending problem. However, we see proportionally more preterm deliveries in women who have an unusually shaped uterus, are carrying more than one baby, have previously delivered early, are smokers, use cocaine or heroin, have had cervical infections during pregnancy (not yeast), or have had unexplained bleeding in the second trimester (not the first). Other factors may be maternal age of less than 18 or more than 40 years, low pre-pregnancy weight, or low socioeconomic status (which often leads to poor health and a lack of proper prenatal care).

THINGS THAT DO NOT CAUSE PRETERM LABOR

There are some widely held but erroneous beliefs surrounding the causes of preterm labor. Here are the facts:

- Intercourse does not cause preterm labor in women who are not susceptible for other reasons.
- Neither does physical stress, although it may cause contractions.
- While many women who deliver early feel that emotional stress was the trigger for preterm labor, scientific studies have failed to reveal a reliable connection between psychological stress and preterm labor. Studies have demonstrated an association of some physically stressful jobs with babies that weigh slightly less, but not to a significant degree.
- Having had one elective first-trimester abortion in a previous pregnancy has not been shown to increase the risk of preterm birth.

GETTING GOOD CARE

At the prenatal visits after 20 weeks, the size of your uterus roughly indicates how the baby is growing, on average increasing a centimeter (about half an inch) a week. At your prenatal appointments, your doctor may measure your tummy as one way to check on your baby. When your practitioner measures from your pubic bone up over the top of your uterus, this translates to about one centimeter for each week of gestation—so at 25 weeks, you will measure 25 centimeters, give or take a few. If your measurements seem too big or too small, your practitioner may do an ultrasound to see if the size of the baby or the amount of amniotic fluid is causing the unexpected measurement. Sometimes everything can be perfectly fine and your baby is simply a little larger or smaller than normal. In other cases, a medical problem may be to blame for the unusual measurements, and further tests may be necessary.

Sometimes it's better to deliver a baby early

Once you start the third trimester, the chances that your baby can thrive outside the womb go up every week. Although the uterus is usually the best place for a fetus until full term, there are situations in which uterine conditions are not so healthy. If the baby starts to show signs of stress, she may be better off being delivered quickly and getting her nutrition and oxygen in the nursery.

How do we know how the baby is doing? In healthy pregnancies, a fetus that is growing well and moving every day is showing us she is OK, and no special monitoring is necessary. In cases where there are risk factors, however—such as a pregnancy that has gone well past the due date (see page 256); a mom who has high blood pressure, long-standing diabetes, or other significant health concerns; or slow growth or other signs that the fetus isn't getting enough nutrients through the placenta—we watch the baby closely using the fetal surveillance tools we have at our disposal. These tools include fetal movement counts (see page 205), non-stress monitoring (page 237), contraction stress tests (page 263), and the biophysical profile (page 265). If these tests are reassuring, the pregnancy can continue without too much worry. If they are questionable, the baby can be watched extra closely, or if she is full term, labor can be induced. If there is a clear-cut problem, even a preterm baby may be delivered because she would be expected to do better outside rather than inside the uterus.

Checking for diabetes of pregnancy

Pregnancy can cause a healthy woman to become temporarily diabetic, a condition known as gestational diabetes, in which hormones from the placenta interfere with the action of insulin, the hormone responsible for the regulation of blood sugar. Gestational diabetes can make a baby grow unusually large, but doctors don't wait for a baby to get too big in order to make a diagnosis. Most practitioners screen all women because there's no way to predict who will develop gestational diabetes, and even when it has no symptoms, the condition can complicate pregnancy. Identifying who has developed diabetes of pregnancy helps the physician protect the fetus from the adverse effects of high maternal blood sugars, which, in rare cases, can even include fetal death. Diabetes testing isn't done until the early third trimester, since many women who will develop gestational diabetes don't get it until late in their pregnancy.

There are two stages of glucose tolerance testing:

- **One-hour glucose testing.** This is a screening test done around 24 to 28 weeks' gestation. Different practitioners use slightly different methods, but the basic concept is that the woman drinks a solution of sugar (glucose) and then, at a specified time interval (often one hour later), gets her blood drawn to check the glucose level. This tests how her body has handled the sugar solution. If the blood sugar level is higher than it should be, more definitive testing is usually needed. Fasting before this test is not required.

- **Oral glucose tolerance testing.** While most diabetic women's one-hour test results will be over the cutoff value and most nondiabetics' results will be under, there is some overlap. The one-hour glucose test really just identifies the group of mothers who need to proceed to the more complicated—and more definitive—oral glucose tolerance test. This test usually requires a three-day special diet (including no food or drink of any kind after midnight the night before the test), followed by drinking a glucose solution. The blood is drawn four times: once before drinking the glucose (when the mother-to-be is fasting); then at one, two, and three hours after consuming the glucose solution. If two or more values are high, gestational diabetes is diagnosed.

Most women with gestational diabetes can be adequately treated with a change in diet, but some will need insulin during pregnancy. Your doctor will give you lots of information if you have diabetes of pregnancy, and will monitor your blood sugars in order to maintain the healthiest environment for your developing baby.

PARENT TO PARENT

"In my 25th week of pregnancy, I was diagnosed with gestational diabetes. I tried to control it with diet and exercise, but it didn't work, so I had to take insulin shots (oh joy, what fun). I had lots of problems—my blood pressure was sky-high, my feet swelled beyond recognition, and I had protein in my urine—girl, I had it going on! I had to have a C-section three weeks early. My point is that, despite all these problems, I'm happy to report that everything went well, and the baby and I are both fine!"

—**misswings,** AS POSTED ON DRSPOCK.COM

Rh sensitization can be prevented
In addition to testing for diabetes in the sixth month, we also make sure to recheck all women who are blood type Rh-negative. (Do you know your blood type? It will

Q: How does Rh immunoglobulin work?

A: An Rh-negative mother will develop antibodies against Rh-positive blood cells (become sensitized) only if fetal blood crosses the placenta and enters her bloodstream. Her immune system then "sees" these cells, identifies them as foreign, and mounts an immune response. The injection of Rh immunoglobulin (RhoGam) blocks the mother's immune system from seeing the fetal cells if they get into her bloodstream, so she will not become sensitized and make antibodies.

RhoGam is given to all Rh-negative women whose fetuses might be Rh-positive. The fetus may be Rh-positive if his father is Rh-positive. If both parents are Rh-negative, they can produce only Rh-negative offspring, and therefore RhoGam is not needed.

RhoGam is given at times during the pregnancy when there is some likelihood of Rh-positive fetal

have been checked at your first prenatal visit and noted in your prenatal chart.)

Blood type is based on particular molecules called antigens that sit on the surface of red blood cells. People have A antigens (type A blood), B antigens (type B), both (type AB), or neither (type O) on their red blood cells. When it comes to Rh factor, some people have

*blood's getting into the mother's bloodstream.
These include:*

. amniocentesis
. miscarriage or ectopic pregnancy
. elective termination of pregnancy
. significant trauma to the abdomen, such as a car accident
. anytime there is bleeding during pregnancy or the practitioner suspects that fetal and maternal blood may have mixed
. around 26 weeks' gestation (which protects through late pregnancy)
. after delivery.

The baby's blood type is checked at birth, using blood obtained from the umbilical cord. If the baby turns out to be Rh-negative as well, the mother's after-delivery dose of RhoGam usually is not necessary.

the Rh antigen (Rh-positive), and some people don't (Rh-negative). In other words, your blood type identifies which antigens you have from each group.

Rh-negative is the only one of these blood groups that can cause a problem during pregnancy. An Rh-negative mother can make antibodies (part of her immune system's response to foreign substances like germs) against Rh-positive blood cells, even against those of her own baby. This is called Rh sensitization. These antibodies have the potential to cross the placenta and attack the fetus's red blood cells, which in turn can cause low blood count (anemia), congestive heart failure, and even fetal death. Fortunately, most Rh sensitization is preventable with an injection of Rh immunoglobulin (RhoGam). Thanks to the development of this drug in 1968, it is now quite rare for an Rh-negative woman to get sensitized and for any related harm to come to her baby. If a woman does develop antibodies against Rh-positive cells, they will be detected in routine pregnancy blood work.

Rh sensitization usually doesn't hurt the baby in the first pregnancy, because the mom can't make enough antibodies to cause severe problems. But the next pregnancy, and any that follow, can become very complicated if a fetus is Rh-positive. If possible, women who become Rh sensitized should get their prenatal care from an obstetrician who is board certified in maternal-fetal medicine and specializes in high-risk cases.

LOOKING AHEAD

Have you been thinking much about labor yet? Some mothers-to-be start worrying about labor and delivery before they even take a pregnancy test, while others don't think much about it until the big day is imminent. Pregnancy is a time of lots of fantasies and fears, and many mothers-to-be even have nightmares about the birth. Be assured that negative dreams and thoughts are *not* premonitions; pregnancy stirs the imagination because so much is at stake and unknowable. One way to channel your concerns is to research the options for your birth experience, and think ahead about your ideal delivery.

Is natural childbirth right for you?

Unmedicated, or so-called natural, childbirth is not for everyone. Many women know ahead of time that they have no interest in the full, primordial experience of giving birth. Natural childbirth can be an incredibly intense experience analogous to running a marathon or climbing a mountain. So why do it? Here are a few reasons to consider:

- Like climbing a mountain, if natural childbirth is a goal you have set for yourself, meeting the challenge (and becoming a mother simultaneously) is a powerful experience, which often gives a tremendous sense of achievement.

- Your experience can be more self-directed and less medical if you avoid an epidural, the most popular form of medicated childbirth (see page 249). An epidural requires an intravenous line (IV), electronic fetal monitoring, and usually bed rest. Without an epidural, if all is going well, you should be able to move around freely or get into a comforting shower or tub. You also may be less likely to require Pitocin (a drug that induces strong contractions; see page 268) or a vacuum or forceps delivery, as well as some other medical procedures. It is as nature intended.

- Women with epidurals are more likely to get a fever in labor, which can sometimes be difficult for the healthcare team to distinguish from infection. This can lead to unnecessary antibiotics for you and for your baby after birth.

There's a strong argument to make for epidurals

If you decide to have an epidural during labor, you're not alone: It's used to relieve pain in childbirth more than any other anesthetic. I'll go into more detail about epidurals and other pain-relieving methods in Chapter 9, but here's a preview so you can start thinking about this popular option:

- An epidural works by distributing small amounts of medication into the nerves around the spinal cord through a small catheter in your back. It generally takes away, or at least diminishes, the pain of contractions. You may lose some feeling in your legs (although you can usually still move them) and probably will have to remain in bed.

- Because an epidural numbs the birth canal, it also can lessen the pain of pushing as the baby descends during delivery. Although the pushing stage may last longer with an epidural, most women still feel the urge to push and are able to do so quite effectively. In some cases, though, the baby may have to be helped out into the world with a special vacuum or forceps (see page 290).

- I have heard people say they don't want an epidural because they don't like the idea that their legs might be weak or numb; they want to be "in control" of their bodies. But if feeling in control is important to you, you may well want an epidural. The emotional experience of unmedicated labor often is anything but controlled, and you may well feel more like yourself during childbirth if you opt for epidural delivery.

Try to keep an open mind

Regardless of your preferences going into labor, it is a good idea to keep an open mind and prepare for whatever comes. Perhaps you've been counting on medicated childbirth but your labor proves to be so rapid that you arrive at the hospital with your cervix dilated eight centimeters and you'll give birth too quickly (or easily). Or maybe there will be numerous emergencies when you arrive at the maternity ward, and anesthesia won't be immediately available. On the other hand, you may be set on natural childbirth but have a long, exhausting labor, and your practitioner determines that your anxiety or fatigue is playing a role in labor's poor progress. She may then recommend an epidural as a treatment to try to get your labor moving. An open mind will help you to reassess the pros and cons of the options, and cope with the unexpected.

Childbirth education classes provide invaluable information

Childbirth education classes are a great tool for helping you learn more about labor and delivery so you can better sort through your options and preferences. Many different types are available: Some (such as The

PARENT TO PARENT

*"I always tell new moms-to-be that there's
no way to predict the pain they'll feel. It
seems to be different for each woman and
every pregnancy. With my first child, I had
very little labor (only 45 minutes) and
absolutely no pain medication. I didn't
need it. With my second, the baby had
trouble getting into position, so they gave
me an epidural. I was petrified, but it was
a godsend. It allowed my muscles to ease
up enough so my son fell right into place
and I delivered 15 minutes later. So go into
labor and delivery with a positive attitude
and half the battle will be won. There is
really nothing to fear, or women wouldn't
keep doing it over and over again!"*

—**dueinJuly,** AS POSTED ON DRSPOCK.COM

Bradley Method or self-hypnosis classes) advocate
particular methods of coping with childbirth and are
aimed at couples who are sure they want an unmedicated, natural birth experience, while hospital-run
classes tend to be more mainstream and medically oriented. Ideally, a class should take a middle-of-the-road

approach, informing the participants about all the different options and letting them decide for themselves which is right for them. When you find a course in tune with your own philosophy, it can help you:

- **Get educated.** You will learn about what physically happens to your body as your baby makes her way into this world.

- **Learn techniques to deal with pain.** The classes will teach you different methods for dealing with contractions. These may include breathing and relaxation exercises, visualization, and comforting activities. Anxiety tends to heighten pain, while peace of mind diminishes it.

- **Feel less fearful and more in control.** Knowledge is power. You will feel less vulnerable if you know exactly what is happening as labor progresses. You will have seen the fetal monitor in class. You will know what the instrument used to break your water looks like. You'll know the normal tests the medical staff will run on your newborn. There will be fewer surprises when the day finally arrives.

- **Be part of a supportive group.** Most classes run over the course of many weeks. You usually get to know the other participants pretty well, and it's comforting to go through the wondrous process of pregnancy and childbirth with others in the same situation. Many classes also hold a reunion session after everyone's given birth, and it can be great fun to swap childbirth stories and see all the babies.

Especially for Dads 🐾

If you're planning on acting as labor coach for your wife or partner (and I seriously hope that you are!), you probably have mixed feelings about this important role. That's only natural—as many as half of all expectant fathers do. Here are some things you can do in the coming months to help prepare for this important step toward parenthood:

- **Educate yourself.** Birth can seem like a pretty mysterious process. Go to the childbirth preparation classes, read a childbirth book specifically geared for dads, maybe even talk with the obstetrician, midwife, or prenatal instructor. There's a good chance that the more that you know about what lies ahead, the more confident you'll feel.

- **Discuss your feelings with your partner.** Your partner needs to know what you're feeling and why, and it can help to find out exactly what she expects from you during labor and delivery. But be particularly sensitive to the way you do this. Instead of being sympathetic, your partner may interpret your apprehensiveness as a sign that you don't care about her or the baby.

- **Clarify your role.** Maybe you like the idea of being there for the birth, but you're concerned about your partner's insistence that you cut the umbilical cord. Or maybe you hate the idea of videotaping the whole blessed event. Yes, this is your wife's big day and you're playing a supporting role, but you still have a right to draw the line at certain things that you're truly reluctant to do. Talk with your partner frankly—she's sure to prefer that you participate in some way, even if it's not exactly on all her own terms.

- **Relax.** No matter how nervous or squeamish you feel anticipating the birth, the reality is that expectant dads rarely fall apart once they're actually in the delivery room. There's something about supporting our wives and wanting to be the first ones to greet our newborns that keeps us relatively calm and focused.

- **Talk to other dads.** Spend some time talking with other men who have stayed with their partner through childbirth. They may have some advice to offer about how they coped with their own squeamishness, for instance, or overcame their feeling of helplessness in the face of their loved ones' pain. Even if they don't have pearls of wisdom to offer, it can be reassuring just to talk things out and get some proof that you're not alone. Most will tell you that being there was a roller-coaster ride of conflicting emotional states, including exhilaration, exhaustion, amazement, boredom, fear, annoyance, panic, and Zenlike calm. And just about all dads will tell you that they wouldn't have missed it for the world.

- **Get additional support.** This may not be a job for one man alone. As a matter of fact, there are few cultures that have only the father providing emotional support to the laboring woman. For millennia, pregnant women in cultures all over the world have gone through labor with another woman at their side. That's the way it used to be here, too. But starting in the 1930s, women began having babies in hospitals instead of at home, and everyone but the woman and her doctors was booted out of the delivery room. In the sev-

Other classes also are available

Childbirth education classes aren't the only ones that may be of interest to you and your partner. Some classes that may be available in your area include:

- early pregnancy
- cesarean birth

enties, dads starting filtering back in, and in 1980, Dr. Marshall Klaus and his colleagues reintroduced the notion of doulas in the U.S. and made the term *doula* a household word. *Doula* (rhymes with *hula*) is actually a Greek word that means "woman caregiver of another woman." Doulas— usually women with children of their own—are thoroughly trained in how to give the laboring mom-to-be *and her husband* (that's you) emotional and physical support throughout labor. She also is a fount of birth-related information, so you'll find you can fire away questions about everything from breech deliveries to Apgar tests. (See page 179 for more on doulas.)

The section above, originally published on drSpock.com, was written by Armin Brott, a nationally recognized parenting expert and author of several best-selling books on fatherhood.

- VBAC (vaginal birth after cesarean)
- breastfeeding
- infant care basics
- infant and child CPR
- baby massage
- sibling classes
- grandparent classes.

Ask your childbirth educator or call your local hospital or birth center to learn about what's offered in your area. When it comes to scheduling, keep in mind that the classes can be all different lengths; some consist of a single session, others run over the course of several weeks. The goal is to have your courses completed around three weeks before your due date. You'll have to pay for most courses, although sometimes scholarships or free classes are available. If money is tight, I usually recommend that parents at least try to take an infant CPR class because it covers such important topics.

NOTES

Use this space to jot down observations about your pregnancy or questions to ask your healthcare practitioner at your next visit:

_____

_____

_____

_____

_____

_____

_____

_____

_____

_____

_____

_____

CHAPTER 7

Weeks 27—31

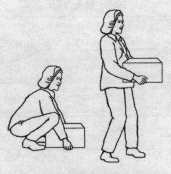

Many moms-to-be experience back pain, but there are things you can do to alleviate the problem. They include using proper form when lifting: Squat, tuck in your buttocks, and hold the object you're lifting close to you. Keep your back straight, and lift using the muscles of your legs. Above all, don't try to pick up anything too heavy!

ABOUT YOUR BABY

Welcome to the third trimester! Your baby's weight is about to triple as she goes from about two pounds at the beginning of this month to seven pounds or so at term. She will take on stores of fat, protein (in the form of muscles and other tissues), calcium (bones), and key nutrients such as iron.

Tucked inside your womb, your child's senses are beginning to develop. She can see light and dark, and she can hear. You may notice that she seems to startle at loud noises or move gently to music.

ABOUT YOU

As you enter this last trimester of pregnancy, your thoughts and dreams are probably taken up with the new arrival and the changes that he will bring to your life and your family. It is time to start thinking about birth and preparing to bring your new baby home. In addition, your body is undergoing a whole new slew of physical changes, which can lead to new—and sometimes annoying—symptoms.

The lowdown on lower-back pain
As the baby grows inside you, your abdomen grows with her; your center of gravity moves forward, and you may find yourself leaning back to compensate. This puts stress on your lower back and is one of the many factors that can lead to back pain in pregnancy. Carrying an extra 30 pounds or more in your middle puts pressure on your back muscles, too, and it doesn't help if your abdominal muscles were a little weak to begin with, as many people's are. To further complicate matters, progesterone is starting to soften the joints of your pelvis, and many women feel a tugging pain where the spine meets the hipbones when they get out of bed or a chair.

With all these elements at work, it's not surprising that most women experience some form of back pain during the course of pregnancy. Here are some simple measures you can take to minimize the discomfort:

- **Start your pregnancy with strong abs.** Going into a pregnancy with strong abdominal muscles can help align the body and decrease the tendency to develop a swayback posture. Unfortunately, though, many of us do not have the foresight to tone up our abs before we get pregnant.

- **Use proper form when lifting.** (See page 164.) Don't bend at the waist. Squat, hold in your buttocks, hold the object you're lifting close to your body, keep your back straight, and lift with your legs. This puts most of the strain on your legs instead of your back. Avoid lifting heavy objects. If you have a young child, try to get him to climb onto you rather than lifting him, when possible.

- **Put your feet up when you can.** Try to take frequent breaks during which you can rest and prop up your feet. If you are required to stand a lot at work, have a footstool or something comparable to rest one foot on while standing; be sure to shift legs from time to time so that the muscles in each get a chance to rest.

- **Sleep on a firm mattress.** You can put a board between your box spring and mattress if your bed is too soft.

- **Assume a comfortable sleep position.** Sleep on your side with your knees bent, and place a pillow between them for support. Another pillow placed under your tummy also may help.

- **Wear low-heeled shoes.** When heels are too high, they push your body forward, putting further pressure on your back.

- **Sit on chairs or couches with good back support.** You also can place a small pillow behind your lower back to help lessen the strain.

- **Use heat to ease back pain.** Place a hot-water bottle or heating pad (wrapped in a towel to avoid burning your skin) on the area where you are having discomfort. Don't slip into a very hot bath instead, because it has the potential to overheat the baby. A *warm* bath, however, is just fine. And don't ever go to sleep while using a heating pad: Such prolonged use could cause burns or even a fire.

- **Get a support belt.** You can buy a special elastic-and-Velcro maternity belt that provides support under your abdomen. You can find one in maternity stores, catalogs, or online.

- **Exercise.** Certain exercises help strengthen your back and improve your flexibility (see page 168). Many women find that the exercises give them relief of pain within a few days or weeks.

A word to the wise: If you are experiencing severe back pain with a fever, if the pain doesn't go away when you rest for a few minutes, or if it occurs when you have a contraction (in which case your uterus will get hard to the touch or feel balled up), call your practitioner. Back pain sometimes can be a sign of a kidney infection or preterm labor.

PREGNANCY EXERCISES FOR YOUR BACK 🐾

*The following exercises are designed to help relieve
the discomfort you may feel as your back tries to
support your expanding belly. They help to stretch
and strengthen the muscles of the back, hips, and
abdomen. Before trying them, I suggest that you
check with your doctor or midwife to be sure that
they're all safe and appropriate in your particular
situation. And remember, especially during
pregnancy, easy does it! Do the exercises slowly, in a
controlled manner, and don't strain.*

Pelvic tilt

- Start on your hands and knees, with your hands
  directly under your shoulders and knees under
  your hips. Your back should be straight, not
  arched. Align your head and neck with your
  straight back.
- Press up with your lower back (like an angry
  cat) and hold for a few seconds. Then relax to
  the straight-back position.
- Do this five times.
- This same exercise may be performed in the
  standing position. Bend your knees, thrust your
  hips slightly forward, and hold your arms out front
  for balance. Then round your back in the angry-cat
  position. Return to the neutral position.

Reverse curl

- Kneel on your hands and knees with your knees 8 to 10 inches apart. Your arms should be straight.
- Come backward slowly tucking your head towards your knees. Keep your hands and arms in the same position. They will now be extended.
- Hold to the count of five, then come back to neutral.
- Do this five times.

Pelvic lifts

- Lie on your back, with your knees bent, your feet on the floor, and your arms at your sides.
- Slowly raise your hips off the floor.
- Slowly lower your hips back to the floor.
- Do this 5 to 10 times. (Note: Lying on your back is OK for short periods of time. Don't stay on your back for more than 5 to 10 minutes.)

Frontward stretch

- Sit in a chair with your back straight. Relax your arms.
- Bend forward slowly so your chest is as close to your knees as possible. Keep your arms dan-

gling forward. If you feel pressure or pain in your abdomen, discontinue this exercise. Hold this position to the count of five.
- Lift your torso up, keeping your back straight.
- Do this five times.

Tabletop bends

- Stand with your legs apart, knees slightly bent, with your hands on your hips.
- Bend forward slowly. Do not arch your back.
- Do this 10 times.

Sciatica often flares up during pregnancy

As your baby grows, your uterus may press on your sciatic nerve, which connects your legs to your spinal cord. Sciatica (sciatic nerve pain) is a sharp or aching pain that usually starts in the lower back or buttocks and sometimes seems to shoot down the back of the leg to the calf or heel.

Most women who experience sciatica notice it first while on their feet. You can try to rest as much as possible to ease the pain. A heating pad or hot-water bottle (wrapped in a towel to avoid burns) applied to the lower back or buttock often alleviates the pain. Back exercises may help with this nagging problem. Sometimes simple leg and lower-back stretches done twice each day can give great relief.

Lower-back stretch

- Stand with your feet 10 to 12 inches apart with your back against a wall.
- Press your lower back into the wall and hold for the count of 10.
- Release.
- Do this 10 times.

Even if sciatica starts fairly early in your pregnancy, you may not be destined to have pain for all the remaining months. Many women grow out of this problem later in pregnancy.

Medical treatment for back pain and sciatica
Acetaminophen (Tylenol) can be an alternative if nothing else seems to be helping. You may want to discuss the use of nonsteroidal medications such as ibuprofen (Motrin, Aleve) with your practitioner to see if they are an option for you. Many physicians believe these medications to be safe until the 32nd week of pregnancy. If the problem gets so severe that you have trouble walking or it is otherwise seriously interfering with your life, discuss treatment options with your practitioner.

❝

PARENT TO PARENT
*"I'm in my third trimester, and I feel as if I
never sleep through the night. As far as
sleep positions are concerned, oddly
enough, one of the ways I'm most
comfortable is partially on my back. I'll
tuck a pillow or the covers under one side
of my body so I'm not completely flat on
my back, and sleep that way. As for not
getting enough sleep, I just try to take
naps whenever I can. I figure that getting
used to this lack of solid sleep may help
in the adjustment period after the baby
is born, anyway."*

—**V0910,** AS POSTED ON DRSPOCK.COM

Getting a good night's sleep can be a challenge
Back pain can interfere with a good night's rest, but
that isn't the only cause of sleep problems in late pregnancy. As your abdomen grows larger, the fetus presses
on your bladder, causing you to make frequent trips to
the bathroom during the night. You may also have
heartburn or an aching in the hips. You may find that
your baby moves more at night, which can keep you

awake. You may have a hard time finding a comfortable position for sleep.

In addition to being uncomfortable, this can be a time of high anxiety. You don't know what to expect regarding labor and delivery. How will you handle the pain? Will the baby be all right when he is born? Will you be ready for the baby? Do you have everything you need? During the day, you may find yourself so tired that you long to go to sleep. When evening finally arrives, you rest for a few hours, then wake up wide-awake. Rest assured that you are not alone: Insomnia during pregnancy is very common.

Here are some tips to help you get some rest before the baby is born and the *real* sleepless nights begin:

- Take a warm bath or shower just before bedtime to start relaxing.
- Before retiring for the night, try a couple of relaxation exercises (you probably learned some in childbirth class).
- Ask your partner for a massage (see page 93).
- Limit the naps you take during the day.
- Get plenty of exercise. A body that works out during the day will be more tired at night. Don't exercise too close to bedtime, though, because you may be too pumped up to go to sleep.
- Clear your mind. Talk with your partner about your worries early in the evening. Try not to focus on your anxieties at night.

- If you are waking up many times during the night to urinate, limit your fluid intake after 4 P.M.

- Avoid caffeine in the late afternoon and evening.

- Make sure that your bedroom is a comfortable temperature. Sleep with the window open or a fan blowing if necessary. (Your partner may need a big blanket to keep him warm.)

- Find a few comfortable positions for sleep. Having many pillows in the bed with you can help. Sleep on your side with your legs bent and a pillow between your legs. Support your abdomen and back with other pillows.

- It's possible that you're hungry. Try a piece of toast or warm milk.

- If you wake up in the middle of the night and can't get back to sleep after a while, don't fret. Get up and do something quiet. Watch television, read, or do needlework until you feel drowsy again. Do your best to try to get to sleep, but don't heap more anxiety on yourself because you're experiencing a bout of insomnia. Resting can be almost as good for you as sleeping. And although it can be frustrating and exhausting, an occasional sleepless night does not damage you or your baby.

Leg cramps can come as an unwelcome surprise

A woman I know told me this story: In her ninth month of pregnancy, she woke up screaming with pain. Her husband sleepily jumped up, grabbed their packed suitcase, and started ushering her off to the hospital.

They were practically out the door before she could make him understand that it wasn't labor, it was a leg cramp!

Indeed, leg cramps can provide some of the most painful episodes of pregnancy. These spasms of the calf muscles, usually lasting a few miserable minutes, can attack anyone at any time, but they are especially common during pregnancy for some unknown reason.

Although calcium, magnesium, potassium, and quinine all have been recommended in the past as prevention for leg cramps, none has been shown to be effective for pregnancy-related cramping. Many moms-to-be find that the cramp begins when they point their toes, so putting a bolster or pillow at the foot of your bed can sometimes be helpful in limiting your leg movements. Some pregnant women find that doing some gentle stretches before going to bed at night helps ward off leg cramps. Once a cramp starts, stretching the calf muscle by flexing the ankle upward and massaging the calf can help diminish the cramp.

As a general rule, leg pain that doesn't go away in a matter of a few hours, or that is accompanied by swelling or difficulty walking, should be evaluated by a doctor.

GETTING GOOD CARE

During the course of your pregnancy and delivery, your healthcare practitioner is likely to recommend several different medical tests or procedures. They might be

TIMELY QUESTIONS

When medical decisions need to be made quickly, it
may be hard to think of all the questions you need to
ask in order to make an informed choice. We have
developed a list to help you think of issues you may
want to discuss with your practitioner in these
situations:

☐ What is my particular problem?

☐ Why is it a problem?

☐ How serious is it?

☐ Describe your suggested treatment.

☐ Why is it necessary (i.e., how will it benefit me or the
baby)?

☐ What are the risks?

☐ Will the treatment resolve my problem completely or just
alleviate it?

something as simple as a blood test or as significant as
a cesarean (see page 209). In an ideal situation, you
would feel complete trust in your doctor or midwife
and her recommendations. She would take care to
explain everything to you without your even asking. In
the real world, however, patients can feel uninformed,

☐ If this doesn't succeed, what will we do next? If this doesn't succeed, what will we do next?

☐ Why does it need to be done now? What happens if we wait a little longer to do it?

☐ What happens if we decide not to do it?

☐ What other alternatives are there?

It is perfectly appropriate to take time to make decisions with your partner or support team. Ask your practitioner to give you some time alone with whomever you want to talk to, even if only for a few minutes. This will help take off some of the pressure and allow you to consult with someone who may be thinking a little more clearly than you are at the time. In some cases, it may be appropriate to ask for a second medical opinion. Remember, your consent is required by law before any medical procedure.

confused, or pressured, especially when a quick decision needs to be made for medical reasons. If you find yourself in this situation, rest assured that you deserve to be an active participant in your own care. Take a proactive role, and keep asking until you get the explanations you need to make informed decisions.

Assemble your childbirth team in advance

Now is a good time to start thinking about the team who will assist you during labor and delivery. "A team?" you may be asking. "All that I'm counting on is the father of my baby's being there." But other people also are available to help you, and their involvement can have a big impact on your childbirth experience.

First, though, let's consider the father of your baby. He is likely to be the key member of your support team. He is the one who knows you best and, of course, he should be there to see his baby come into the world. There isn't anything in the backgrounds of most American men, however, that prepares them to provide support for a woman in labor. And even in other cultures where it's traditional for men to play some role during childbirth, it is rare for the father of the baby to be the sole support for the laboring woman. Both you and your husband or partner probably could use a little additional help and guidance.

STAYING IN TOUCH

As your due date draws closer, it's important to be able to reach your partner at all times, even if it means getting a beeper or cell phone. If you don't already have one, check with your local hospital— some have reasonably priced "baby beeper" rental programs for expectant families.

Obstetrical nurses can be a great help

If you're giving birth at a hospital or some birth centers, your support team automatically will include a registered nurse who will be assigned to you when you are admitted. She will have completed nursing school and passed state board licensing examinations. In addition to providing medical care to you during childbirth, she may function as a labor coach in conjunction with your spouse or partner. These nurses are usually kind, competent, and experienced, but they often have a number of patients assigned to them and may not be able to stay at your side the way your partner or doula will. You also probably won't be able to choose which nurse is assigned to you, and there can be a clash in your outlooks; some nurses are very supportive of natural childbirth, while others are more active advocates of epidurals and other medical pain-relieving measures.

Doulas can be a mother's best friend

Research indicates that having a female team member to provide emotional and practical support in labor can shorten the length of labor and decrease the need for pain medications, Pitocin (see page 268), and other interventions, including a cesarean section. Your nurse may not be able to take on this role, due to her other responsibilities. You may want to invite a female friend or relative to accompany you, especially if they have childbirth experience and have a calming influence on you. Or you can hire your own professional labor assistant, or doula.

A doula is a woman trained in the emotional and physical support of women in labor. Doulas do not provide medical care to women in labor, and do not deliver babies. Some are certified by a well-known organization, Doulas of North America (DONA). Most doulas will meet the family before the birth, talk about the birth plan, and then be there for the family through labor and birth, and sometimes beyond. Studies have shown that women attended by doulas have lower cesarean rates and use fewer epidurals than women with traditional labor support. One common misconception: Doulas do *not* undercut fathers during delivery. A study on the involvement of the fathers in doula-supported labors showed the same or more contact between the parents compared with labors in which the fathers were the only coaches. In addition, a lot of dads-to-be find that having a doula takes the pressure off them and allows them to fully experience the process of becoming a father. To get more information, contact Doulas of North America at *www.dona.org*.

Many nurse-midwives provide professional labor support as well as medical care during labor and birth. If you are going to a nurse-midwife, ask her about whether there would be value in hiring a doula, or if she will provide the same kind of help.

No matter whom you enlist in your labor-support team and how carefully you stack the deck to have the kind of experience you want, keep in mind that you can't always control the events of labor and delivery. No one can promise you it will be exactly as you dream it to be—actually, it is pretty likely to be quite different from the way you imagine, especially if you're a first-time mom. However, you might as well do your part to make it the best experience that you can. So think ahead about your priorities, and try to find a good balance between being open-minded and accepting the unexpected while setting the scene to support what is important to you.

LOOKING AHEAD

As I've said before, the more you learn about the routine—and even some of the not-so-routine—events of labor, the more likely you'll be to feel at least somewhat in control and to make good decisions when your time comes. There's nothing more terrifying than going into childbirth not understanding what is happening to your body and your child, and what the medical staff might do to help you along. Here, and in the next few chapters, I'll explain about these events to reinforce what you're probably already learning in your childbirth-preparation classes. We'll begin with the phases of labor.

Labor usually follows a predictable path
Most people think of labor and delivery as being one single process, but there are actually a few distinct phases. Particularly if you have chosen to have an unmedicated birth, you will most likely go through predictable emotional and physical changes that are characteristic of each phase as your cervix (the opening to your uterus) fully dilates to 10 centimeters, so you can push out your baby.

THE PROS AND CONS OF DOULAS 🐾

Q: *I am thinking about getting a doula. But when I mentioned it to my OB/GYN, she wrinkled her nose. My sister used a doula and had a wonderful experience, and I am intrigued. Can you explain a little about the pros and cons?*

A: I have to preface this by saying that I am a doula fan. That said, I recognize that there are points to be made on both sides of the issue.

Cons: Some practitioners (like your OB) have had negative experiences with doulas. Many doulas are strongly (some might even say militantly) supportive of natural, unmedicated childbirth, and may be viewed by the hospital staff as preventing the woman from getting "her" epidural. In these cases, doctors and nurses may see a doula as working against what they consider the best interests of their patient, or they may resent her interference with normal hospital practices.

Pros: The doula can be your advocate in the hospital: She's there to make sure that your wishes are carried out if at all possible. She knows comfort measures for labor and can help alleviate pain without resorting to medication, if that's the type of birth you've chosen. The doula also supports your partner and keeps him involved in the process.

- **Pre-labor.** Before labor, and often in early labor, many women feel an urge that is sometimes called nesting. This usually involves activities such as cleaning, decorating, buying baby clothes or supplies, or doing other tasks that make your home more ready for a baby. Some women who have already had a few children are able to use this urge as a marker for getting close to delivery, while others have nesting urges on and off in the third trimester.

- **Stage 1: Latent Phase (zero to about 4 centimeters dilated).** Latent phase is the part of labor when you feel most like yourself. Your contractions may be painful, but you can manage, and in between contractions you are able to relax.

- **Stage 1: Active Phase (from about 4 centimeters until fully dilated).** During active phase, your contractions are more frequent and more intense. You may find it more difficult to relax and may need your coach to help you to keep focused. When possible, water therapy in the form of a shower or bath can be helpful at this time. Many women also are more comfortable when they move around.

- **Stage 1: Transition (about 8 to 9 centimeters dilated, sometimes less).** Transition occurs just before it is time to push. If labor is very rapid, you can find yourself in transition at 5 or 6 centimeters, but usually it starts around 8 or 9. Transition is the most emotionally challenging part of labor. Thankfully, it is also usually the shortest. Transition is often characterized by a feeling of panic or discouragement. This is the time many women feel that they cannot cope and ask for medications. It is crucial for your coach to understand the normalcy of your feelings, and how short is the time you will be feeling this bad. The end is in sight!

- **Stage 2: Pushing.** You will have reached complete dilation and feel the urge to push. Usually you'll experience a sense of relief and some pleasure in taking a more active role. The intense feelings of transition have abated, and you can focus on the work ahead. Some women develop pain as the baby's head descends, but take comfort that you can see the finish line and soon will have the baby in your arms.

- **Birth.** I don't have words to describe the range of feelings that new parents have at the moment of birth. One moment all you can focus on is how overwhelmed you feel and how much you want labor to be over. Then, all of a sudden, the stress is gone and the baby is there. You are flooded with happiness and wonderment at the miracle that you and your partner produced.

- **Stage 3: Delivery of the placenta.** A few minutes after the baby is born, your body will expel the placenta. This is usually painless and easy. In fact, you may not be paying too much attention to this part, since your baby will probably be taking your mind off everything else.

Tracking the progress of your labor

While you're going through the phases of labor, your midwife, OB/GYN, or other birth attendant will monitor your progress on a regular basis to see how close you are to giving birth. She'll do so mainly by performing periodic cervical exams with her gloved, lubricated fingers (not the speculum). By the third trimester you'll probably have had at least one cervical exam, so you'll have a good idea of what it will feel like. Exams during labor are usually done with you lying on your back in a bed, with your knees bent and apart. Although prenatal exams often involve the use of stirrups, once you're in labor, you often can just rest your feet on the bed with your legs drawn up.

As with any internal examination, taking slow, deep breaths can help to relax the vaginal muscles. The more you're able to relax, the easier it is for your practitioner to reach the cervix, which may be located high up inside the vagina in early labor. Some women find the exam painful, while others find it merely a little uncomfortable. During labor, many mothers-to-be want to find out about their progress, so they actually may look forward to the exam.

Your practitioner may use some unfamiliar terms to describe your progress

The following is a list of definitions of some terms you may hear from your practitioner as she reports the changes in your cervix:

- **Cervical ripening.** Early in labor, or even at a late prenatal visit, your practitioner may tell you that your cervix is ripe. This means that your cervix has softened (a cervix earlier in pregnancy typically feels similar to a nose and later becomes more like an earlobe) and may be even somewhat dilated (opened) or effaced (shortened). *Ripeness* is a term sometimes used to indicate that your body is ready for labor.

- **Dilation.** This term applies to the width that the cervix is open. Dilation can begin before labor actually starts or in early labor, and is measured in centimeters. For most deliveries, the cervix needs to dilate to 10 centimeters before pushing can begin and the baby delivered. This range is based on the fact that a full-term baby's head is about 10 centimeters across.

- **Effacement.** This is the shortening of the cervix, sometimes referred to as *thinning out*. Like dilation, it begins before or during early labor. Before effacement takes place, the cervix is like a long bottleneck, usually about four centimeters (almost two inches) in length. The cervix then shortens, or effaces, pulling up into the uterus and becoming part of the lower uterine wall. Effacement may be measured in percentages, from 0 percent (not effaced at all) to 100 percent, which describes a paper-thin cervix.

- **Station.** This term refers to how low the baby is in the pelvis. Station is determined by feeling where the baby rests in relation to the mother's ischial spines, the parts of the pelvic bones that protrude slightly in toward the birth canal and can be felt inside the vagina by an experienced examiner. *Minus-5 station* means the baby is floating above the pelvis, about five centimeters above the ischial spines. *Zero station* means the baby has dropped or engaged well into the pelvis and that his head rests right at the level of the ischial spines. And *plus* 5 means the baby's head not only has come down about 5 centimeters past the ischial spines, but also is visible at the opening of the vagina (also known as crowning).

The exams may be more uncomfortable at first

Near the beginning of labor, cervical exams may be a bit more uncomfortable than they will be as labor progresses, because the practitioner may have to reach fairly high into the vagina to check the cervix. This often happens, in part, because the baby's head has not yet dropped deep into the pelvis, bringing the cervix closer to the vaginal opening. This is normal.

As labor advances, the cervix will move around to the front and become much more accessible, making the exams more comfortable. In the latent phase of labor, the cervix will typically dilate to four centimeters so that the opening is about the size of a silver dollar. By the end of this phase, effacement is usually 100 percent.

The cervix during the active phase

Generally, when the cervix has dilated four to five centimeters, a woman is considered to be in active labor, and faster progress in terms of cervical dilation is typically made for each hour of contractions.

The cervix will continue to dilate to 10 centimeters. During this time, there may be a slight to moderate amount of bleeding from the cervix. The mother may start to feel more pelvic pressure and may even feel the urge to push as the baby moves lower into the birth canal. If she isn't fully dilated, it's important for her to resist the urge to push, because in some instances the cervix will tear.

This phase of labor also includes the transition phase, which typically begins when the cervix is about 8 centimeters dilated and continues until 10 centimeters. When you reach complete dilation in your own labor, it will be time for the real action to begin—when you can begin to bear down and push out the little miracle you've been waiting so long to meet.

NOTES

Use this space to jot down observations about your pregnancy or questions to ask your healthcare practitioner at your next visit:

_____

_____

_____

_____

_____

_____

_____

_____

_____

_____

_____

_____

CHAPTER 8

Weeks 32–35

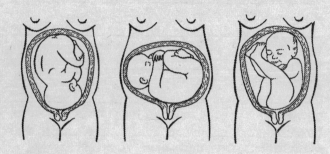

By the middle of the third trimester, your baby is likely to have settled into the headfirst, or cephalic, position (baby on the left). However, some babies are still in the breech position (baby on the right), with their feet or buttocks poised to be born first. And a few babies have assumed the transverse-lie position (baby in the middle), in which they are stationed sideways in the uterus. By 40 weeks, however, more than 95 percent of babies will move themselves into the headfirst position.

ABOUT YOUR BABY

You are now at the time of pregnancy when your fetus will be doing some things that you probably think of as real-live baby activities. Inside your womb, he is moving his arms and legs, swallowing amniotic fluid to exercise his digestive system, urinating, and sucking his thumb. He goes through the motions of breathing, allowing amniotic fluid to move in and out of his lungs. You may even notice an occasional rhythmic jostling or jumping that indicates a bout of fetal hiccups. In short, he is practicing for life in the outside world.

As you feel him move about, you're sure to take comfort in these tangible signs that he's doing well. Your instincts are well founded: One way that medical professionals evaluate fetal condition is to follow how much a baby is moving (see page 205). As a general rule, a baby is in good condition if he moves at least 10 times during three different time periods each day. Most babies move much more than that (as you're probably well aware by now!).

Your baby's kicks can provide clues to her position

When you feel your baby move, do you wonder about how she is positioned in your uterus? Often, a pregnant woman feels the most fetal movement where the baby's feet are. If you feel kicks near the top of your uterus, the baby is more likely to be headfirst—that is, upside down in the womb. This is the best position (your doctor or midwife may also use the term *presentation*) for delivery because the head is the largest part of a baby, and once that fits through the birth canal, the rest is generally smooth sailing. If the kicks are all down low, she may be breech (buttocks or feet first). A few are in an even rarer position: sideways in the uterus, known as the transverse-lie position. In this case, the kicks can be felt anywhere in the abdomen.

By the middle of the third trimester, a fetus in the headfirst, or cephalic, presentation usually stays that way because her head fits so nicely into her mother's pelvis. Breech or transverse-lie babies, on the other hand, usually continue to change positions. Eventually, most turn headfirst and settle in. By 38 weeks, more than 95 percent of babies are in the cephalic position, 3 to 4 percent are breech, and a few are transverse. Most breech babies and all transverse babies have to be delivered by cesarean section.

If you can't tell how your baby is positioned, your practitioner may be able to figure it out by examining your abdomen. A baby's head feels hard and round and moves separately from her back. A baby's butt also can feel pretty hard, though, so sometimes the practitioner still can't know for sure; a vaginal examination done late in the pregnancy often can provide a better idea. Even if the mother's cervix is closed, the lower part of the uterus may be thin enough to feel the bones of a baby's skull (or the chubbiness of the buttocks) through it.

Usually a practitioner will try to determine the position of the fetus by 35 to 37 weeks, to see if anything needs to be done to help the baby rotate before birth. If the examination is inconclusive, ultrasound can give a definitive answer. If the baby is in the wrong position, you can try several procedures to encourage her to rotate (see page 206).

Q: I am pregnant with my third child. My first was delivered vaginally with no complications. My second was delivered vaginally in the breech position. Ultrasounds of this third baby show that he also is in the breech position, and large for his gestational age. The doctor tried to turn my second child into the headfirst position, but the baby was too big. At what point is it safe to try to turn this third baby into the headfirst position before he also gets too big?

A: Even though doctors might be more successful turning babies into the headfirst position earlier in pregnancy, we don't usually like to try until around 36 or 37 weeks. In the rare case in which there is a complication during the procedure and the child needs to be delivered right away, we don't want to end up delivering a preemie. I understand that you're worried about your baby getting too big, but the good news is that it's usually not the size of the baby that prevents a successful version. Rather, the exact position of the baby and whether or not he already has engaged in the mother's pelvis are more important. The fact that this is your third child works in your favor; the more babies a woman has had, the less likely the baby is to have dropped into position by 36 weeks.

ABOUT YOU

You are heading into the homestretch of pregnancy, and
may be riding a roller coaster of emotions. One minute
you may be very excited to meet your new son or daugh-
ter, then suddenly feel extremely worried whether or not
your baby will be healthy. You may fret that you don't
know enough to be a good mother, but then become
convinced that you and the baby's father are going to be
the best parents ever. You also may be very apprehensive
about the birth, and how well you and your partner will
perform. In addition to this strong surge of emotions,
physical changes continue in the third trimester, and
many of them can be uncomfortable and sometimes
even embarrassing. In this section we will talk about
some of the less pleasant (OK, downright icky) changes
of the third trimester: bladder problems, constipation,
hemorrhoids, varicose veins, skin changes (including
itchy rashes), clumsiness, and confusion.

Bladder problems may send you scurrying for the bathroom

You may feel as if your bladder is about the size of a
walnut—and it may well be. As the baby grows larger,
there's less room in your abdominal cavity for your
bladder. You probably are finding that you have to urinate frequently, just as you did in early pregnancy. You
may also lose a small amount of urine when you
sneeze, cough, or abruptly change position, a condition
known as stress urinary incontinence (SUI). Sometimes
SUI is a mild and infrequent event, and sometimes it
can be severe, interfering with normal activities.

SUI is very common in pregnancy and the postpartum period. In pregnancy, there is pressure on the bladder from the enlarging uterus. Trauma to the nerves and muscles of the pelvic floor during childbirth can worsen stress incontinence postpartum. Often the symptoms will resolve within a few months after the baby is born, even without any treatment. Kegel exercises strengthen the pelvic-floor muscles, allowing better urinary control. The exercises are easy to do, but you must rack up about 100 to 200 Kegels a day to see a difference in urinary control! If loss of urine continues, consult your practitioner to discuss treatment options.

HOW TO DO KEGELS

If you lose a little urine when you sneeze or change positions, these exercises, named after the doctor who devised them, will help you maintain better urinary control. And even if you're not yet showing any symptoms, it's still a good idea to learn how to do Kegels to help your body recover from the physical stress that delivery wreaks on your pelvic muscles.

The easiest way to understand which muscles of the pelvic floor you need to contract is to sit on the toilet and practice starting and stopping the flow of urine. Once you have identified which muscles to use, however, it's best not to do these exercises while you're urinating; otherwise, you might not empty your bladder completely. While you're doing your Kegels, be sure to keep your back, abdominal, and thigh muscles relaxed so you can concentrate on your pelvic-floor muscles.

- Concentrate on pulling your pelvic muscles up and in.

Pregnancy is a constipating affair

Ironically, while it can be a little too easy to urinate, many pregnant women find that they have the opposite problem when it comes to another aspect of waste elimination. In advanced pregnancy, your big uterus

- In the beginning, hold the contraction of the muscles to the count of three.
- Relax to the count of three.
- Repeat this contraction-relaxation pattern 10 times.
- Do a set of Kegels at least five times a day.
- As your muscles get stronger, work up to holding each contraction to the count of 10 and increasing the number of repetitions to 20 per set.

Yes, these are a lot of Kegels, but once you get the hang of the exercises, you can perform them anywhere—sitting in your car at a stoplight, watching television, even doing the dishes. Sometimes earmarking certain activities as Kegel time can help you remember to do them; consider doing Kegels every time you talk on the phone, wait in line, or watch ads on TV. Be consistent. You'll see the best results if you do them every day. And be patient: It can take about six weeks or so before you notice a marked improvement.

pressing on the intestines adds to the constipation you already may have been having from hormones, supplemental calcium, and prenatal vitamins. After the baby comes, if there is pain from sutures or swelling at the opening of your vagina, you may feel afraid to have a bowel movement, and consciously or unconsciously hold back. Narcotic pain medications (such as codeine) also are constipating.

Constipation can be quite a problem throughout pregnancy and the postpartum period; for many women, it becomes a lifelong struggle. Still, there are ways to ward off or alleviate the condition. For example, you can:

- Exercise regularly.
- Drink plenty of liquids.
- Increase your fiber intake. Eat fiber-rich foods such as fruits, vegetables, and high-fiber cereals. Even with a healthy, balanced diet, your fiber intake may not be adequate. Try psyllium fiber supplements like Metamucil or Citrucel. Although you may think of them as laxatives, they are simply a concentrated source of fiber, and therefore safely serve a useful purpose. The powder forms work better than tablets for most people. Be sure to drink a lot of liquids. Fiber supplements are safe even if taken on a daily basis.
- Pick a time of day to routinely try to move your bowels. Many people find that trying to have a BM after breakfast or after a cup of coffee is better than waiting until they feel the urge. Rushing around all day, ignoring the mild signals you get from your body, is not conducive to normal bowel function.
- Medications can help. Stool softeners (Colace and generic versions) and mild laxatives like milk of

magnesia are safe to use during pregnancy. Milk of magnesia also can be used for heartburn. It is always best to avoid stimulant laxatives (such as Dulcolax and Ex-Lax) unless directed by your practitioner. If you are not sure about a laxative's safety, be sure to ask your doctor or midwife.

Hemorrhoids are a common problem

Hemorrhoids are varicose veins that sit just inside or outside the anal opening. These swollen, enlarged blood vessels lie just under the surface of the skin and can lead to irritation of the skin and, occasionally, bleeding with bowel movements.

Two factors contribute to hemorrhoids in pregnancy. The uterus puts pressure on the veins that bring blood back from the lower body to the heart; at the same time, the pregnancy hormone progesterone relaxes the walls of the veins. This combination causes the veins in the lower half of the body to swell. Gravity also plays a role if you stand or sit for long periods of time. Constipation adds to these factors, setting the scene for severe (though probably temporary) hemorrhoid problems.

To help prevent or lessen problems from hemorrhoids:

- Avoid getting constipated, and try not to push or strain when you are having a bowel movement. Of course, during a vaginal birth, you have to push out your baby, and your hemorrhoids may temporarily get worse.

- If you do become constipated, treat it before it gets severe.

- Topical therapy of hemorrhoids can give relief of symptoms. You can use over-the-counter creams, ointments, and suppositories that contain hydrocortisone to soothe the inflammation. You can sit in warm water in your bathtub or in a plastic sitz-bath tub that fits into your toilet (sitz baths can be purchased at drugstores). The warm water is very soothing and can help clean the area if it is too painful to wipe. You also can use pads containing witch hazel, an astringent solution (under the brand name Tucks), which can be purchased over the counter. These are used for cleansing and soothing the hemorrhoid area.

For most women, hemorrhoids are a temporary nuisance. But on rare occasions, if a large clot forms in the dilated vein, surgery is needed. These clots are very painful, but the surgical procedure to remove them is relatively minor. The procedure is done with local anesthesia in the office or hospital.

Varicose veins can make your legs swell and ache

Hemorrhoids aren't the only type of varicose veins women get in pregnancy. As your growing uterus places increased pressure on the circulation system in your lower body, blood flow can slow down. In some women, blood pools in certain veins where gravity's pull is the greatest. This may result in one or more bulging, bluish, itchy, achy veins. They usually occur in the legs, but they also can develop near the opening of the vagina. Varicose veins tend to run in families, and many women first notice them during pregnancy. With subsequent pregnancies, varicose veins tend to get worse.

Unfortunately, there is no way to prevent varicose veins, but there are a few things you can do to help reduce the swelling and soreness you may experience, and prevent them from becoming worse:

- Wear support hose (both department-store and prescription types are available, depending upon the severity of your problem).
- Avoid long periods of uninterrupted sitting or standing. When sitting, elevate your legs above the level of your hips as often as possible.
- Exercise regularly.
- Don't sit with your legs crossed.
- Don't wear socks or knee-high stockings with a tight elastic band at the top.
- Avoid excessive weight gain.

Typically, a few months after delivery, most of the symptoms associated with your varicose veins will go away, although the veins themselves will likely remain. If their appearance or discomfort continues to bother you, ask your doctor about treatment options.

Yet more skin changes may occur
As if varicose veins, constipation, and hemorrhoids weren't enough, you may notice annoying skin changes

during pregnancy, which we started to discuss in Chapter 4. Small, dilated capillaries called spider veins, skin tags, and other skin changes are common. Most of these are normal, although they may not totally resolve after the baby is born. Any change in a mole or the development of an irregular freckle or bump always deserves to be checked by a healthcare professional.

Itchy skin is also a common problem in pregnancy, especially on the abdomen. While this may be just due to your skin's getting dry as it stretches, a common cause of itching is PUPPPs (if you *have* to know: pruritic [itchy] urticarial [hivelike] papules [little bumps] and plaques [bigger bumps] of pregnancy). PUPPPs can be treated with lotions containing hydrocortisone or, when necessary, stronger medications. If you are suffering from itchy bumps on your abdomen, chest, arms, or legs, ask your doctor or midwife what to do.

Your belly button changes

Speaking of your abdomen, you may have noticed that as it expands, your navel—the scar from where your umbilical cord was attached to your mother—gets stretched. Even if you have a deep belly button (or innie) when not pregnant, you may find that first your navel flattens and then eventually protrudes from your abdomen. This doesn't bother some women, while others find it annoying to have a bump on an already large tummy. A band-aid across the area can make it less noticeable through your clothing. (A woman I know told me that she felt like the turkey she got for Thanksgiving: When her belly button popped out, she figured the baby

Q: This is my second pregnancy and I am dealing with a problem that just about made me crazy the first time around! All over my belly, I have little bumps that itch worse than mosquito bites. My stomach is covered with scabs from scratching. All this started at about 35 or 36 weeks in my first pregnancy, but it happened even earlier this time. Please help.

A: You've described a skin condition called PUPPPs. Unfortunately, it does tend to recur in subsequent pregnancies, and, as you well know, it can be miserable. Many mothers-to-be get relief with topical steroid creams, such as those that contain hydrocortisone, and with mildly sedating antihistamines, such as Benadryl. Talk to your doctor about your rash, and see what treatment she recommends for you.

was done! Although it would be nice if such a clear-cut sign existed, the two events are not related, of course.)

You may feel clumsy or confused

Many women feel clumsy or foggy-headed during pregnancy. Some of it may be caused by distraction— thinking about how you are feeling or about your baby-to-be—or maybe by poor sleep. Ultimately, the causes of these annoying problems aren't known, but they are common enough to be worth mentioning, if only to reassure you that these experiences are normal and will resolve after the baby is out.

THE SILVER LINING 🐝

While the third trimester can be one of the more uncomfortable periods of pregnancy, it is also one of the most exciting. If you are getting frustrated with your aches and pains as well as the changes in your shape, keep in mind that you are accomplishing an amazing feat: You are growing a whole person inside your body. Try to keep a good attitude and recognize that the discomfort is temporary. You are almost there. Your little one will come out soon to meet you!

GETTING GOOD CARE

In the eighth month, your prenatal visits are usually scheduled at two-week intervals. Your doctor or midwife needs to check your blood pressure, the growth of the baby, and how both of you are faring. Often, a mother has lots of questions as childbirth draws closer, and these more frequent visits give you a chance to ask for information and share your thoughts.

There are times when it is important to watch the baby extra closely to be sure he is doing well. This usually occurs in high-risk pregnancies, as with maternal hypertension or diabetes, or if the baby isn't growing well. And if the mother goes past her due date, we need to monitor the situation carefully to be sure the placenta is still supplying the fetus with an adequate amount of oxygen and nutrients.

Your doctor may recommend fetal-movement counts

As I mentioned earlier in this chapter, fetal movement is an important indicator of a baby's health and well-being. Usually a mother's general impression that the baby is moving normally, backed up by her practitioner's observations during the prenatal visits, is enough to indicate that the baby is in good condition. Sometimes, though, a practitioner may think that a more formal and accurate accounting is warranted and initiates fetal-movement counts (also known as kick counts).

If your doctor recommends this in your case, he'll ask you to keep a chart of how much the baby moves every day after meals (babies tend to be most active just after their mothers eat). You'll mark down all the movements you feel in, say, half an hour, or how long it takes to feel 10 movements (different doctors may use different protocols). If the baby hasn't moved at least 10 times, you'll continue to count for a full hour, lying on your side, which helps you pay attention and may improve the blood flow to the baby. Most babies will keep to the same pattern of movements during the day. If the baby isn't moving, or moves much less than usual, you should call your practitioner to see what to do next. Most of the time, he'll have you come to the office or hospital for electronic fetal monitoring or ultrasound.

Several approaches can coax your baby into the headfirst position

Before 35 weeks, your practitioner won't be too worried about your baby's not being in the proper position for childbirth (see page 190). But if a breech or transverse-lie baby doesn't turn on her own in the ninth month, your doctor or midwife might try helping her get into the headfirst position. For example, your practitioner might have you get into a position that encourages the baby to turn. Lying head down on your back on a slant board (or a sturdy ironing board carefully placed at an angle against a bed) can help the baby dislodge from your pelvis and flip into the headfirst position. Never try this without having someone spot for you or without the recommendation of your practitioner. Most doctors or midwives recommend trying this for five minutes a few times a day.

Your practitioner also might borrow a page from Eastern medicine and suggest that you try moxabustion, the technique of burning a Chinese herb at a specified point on one of your toes. It may sound unusual, but scientific studies have shown that moxabustion can help a breech baby move into a headfirst position. Typically, a trained acupuncturist would be needed for this treatment.

More commonly, your doctor will recommend a medical procedure called external cephalic version, or simply version, for short. The doctor pushes on the baby through the mother's abdomen, either creating a forward roll like a somersault or a back flip. Ultrasound is usually used to watch the baby and determine if the rotation has been successful. The success rate for rotating a baby to headfirst position is quoted as being anywhere between 35 and 86 percent, and research has shown that offering version to all mothers with breech babies at 36 weeks' gestation decreases the cesarean rate for that group of women. The procedure is more successful in women who have had other children (since the baby can move around more easily) than it is for a first-time mom. It also works better if the baby is small, the amniotic fluid is plentiful, and the baby's bottom hasn't already settled into the mother's pelvis. Often, a medication that suppresses contractions is given to relax the uterus before version is done.

The baby's heart rate sometimes will slow during or immediately after version, especially when it is successful. The heart rate usually comes back to normal within a few moments, and there is no evidence that this short-lived slowdown harms the baby in any way. In very rare situations, the heart rate stays slow long enough that practitioners will start the initial preparations for an emergency cesarean section. Although preparation is sometimes necessary, actual emergency cesareans are extremely rare under these circumstances.

While it's very unusual to have a serious complication of external version, it can be uncomfortable or even moderately painful. Some physicians offer epidurals to eliminate pain and totally relax the abdominal muscles, which makes the procedure more likely to succeed. Your doctor will tell you what options are available at your hospital. If you undergo this procedure, remember that you always have the right to stop it for any reason. (It's your body, after all!) Ideally, you will want a support person with you during version, and you'll need someone to drive you home from the hospital.

If the baby settles into the headfirst position, you'll probably go home for a while to await the natural onset of labor. If the baby fails to turn, your doctor is likely to schedule a cesarean in the near future.

There is some controversy over whether it's OK to do external cephalic version on a woman who has had a prior cesarean, but studies have not shown an increased rate of complications in this group. The only real argument not to try version is if you know you will need a C-section for some other reason.

GROUP B STREP TESTING

During a prenatal visit towards the end of the third trimester, you may be tested for Group B streptococcus (also called GBS). This is a type of bacterium that lives in the vaginal region and skin of about 15 percent of women. It does no harm to the women, but in rare instances it can cause serious illnesses (such as pneumonia, meningitis, or bloodstream infections) in newborns if it is transmitted during delivery.

The test involves placing a cotton swab into the vagina or rectum. The swab then is sent to the lab to see if this particular bacterium is present. If your GBS test is positive, you will be given antibiotics during labor to prevent transmission to your baby during birth (taking antibiotics before labor is not recommended).

LOOKING AHEAD

This is the time in pregnancy to get educated about all the "what-ifs." One of the big what-ifs looming on your childbirth horizon might be the possibility of a cesarean section instead of a standard vaginal delivery. Even if there's no reason to suspect that you might need a cesarean, things can happen at the last minute, and learning about this common operation can help you get ready for any eventuality. Understanding the possibilities can help you feel more secure and allow you to be a more active participant in your own care. Thinking about C-section ahead of time also gives you a chance to ask questions about your practitioner's attitudes toward cesarean sections, the hospital's cesarean rate, and general hospital routines.

What is a cesarean section?

A cesarean birth, or C-section, can involve anything from a scheduled operation planned well in advance to an unexpected emergency. It can mean severe disappointment for a mother who had her heart set on a vaginal delivery, or it can come as a welcome relief after a long and difficult labor.

In a cesarean, the baby is born through surgical incisions in her mother's abdomen and uterus. Cesareans require two incisions: one through the abdominal wall and one into the uterus. The skin incision is usually a "bikini" incision across the lower abdomen, but in some circumstances a vertical incision from the belly button down to the pubic hair is made instead. The uterine incision is usually a low-transverse incision (across the stretchy portion of the lower uterus), allowing the woman to labor in the future without great risk of uterine rupture.

There are several situations in which a cesarean might be necessary:

- **The baby isn't fitting through the birth canal.** A large baby, a mother's small pelvis, or poor contraction strength may result in this impasse. The most common cause, however, is a slight change in the baby's position, so that he presents a larger diameter of his head to the birth canal and doesn't fit through (if his head's tipped to the side, for example). This explains why a woman can need a cesarean for one baby and, subsequently, fit an even larger baby through the birth canal without problems. You may hear your doctor use the technical terms for the reasons in this category, such as failure to progress in labor, arrested active phase, failure of descent, or cephalopelvic disproportion (CPD).

- **Placenta previa.** This condition occurs when the placenta, instead of implanting along the front, back, or top portion of the uterus, lies across the internal opening of the cervix, blocking the baby's path. It may be diagnosed during a routine ultrasound, or if there is vaginal bleeding in the second or third trimester. If the placenta continues to cover the cervical opening (also called the cervical os), a cesarean is necessary to safely deliver the baby.

- **Previous cesarean.** There was a time when doctors lived by the dictum "Once a cesarean, always a cesarean." When that rule was established, cesareans were less common and involved a large vertical incision in the uterus that created a weak spot right where the contractions were strongest. The risk of uterine rupture (the scar in the uterus popping open) during a subsequent pregnancy was significant.

Nowadays, most cesareans are done crosswise, in the lower, less contractile part of the uterus. In these low-transverse cesareans, the risk of uterine rupture is greatly reduced, and most physicians believe that vaginal birth after cesarean (VBAC) is a safe option—maybe even safer than a repeat cesarean. Note that the type of incision in the skin may not go the same direction as the incision in the uterus, and it is the *uterine* incision that determines the risk of uterine rupture. The surgical note or the word of the surgeon is the best way to determine what type of cesarean you had.

- **The baby isn't coming headfirst.** As mentioned earlier, breech babies are often delivered by cesarean section, and transverse-lie babies always are (they just can't fit through the birth canal sideways). In both situations, a cesarean avoids the risk of cord prolapse, in which the umbilical cord, which brings oxygen to the fetus, precedes the baby into the birth canal. As the baby follows, his weight could pinch off the flow of blood— and therefore oxygen—through the cord.

- **Infections in the birth canal.** A cesarean is often performed to protect the baby if the mother has active genital herpes, or other infections like human immunodeficiency virus (HIV), which can be transmitted during delivery. A previous history of herpes is not a reason for a cesarean as long as there is no current outbreak. Some women who know that they have herpes take medications toward the end of pregnancy to prevent an outbreak so that they don't have to have a cesarean. If a woman's partner has herpes and she doesn't, they should talk to the practitioner about what steps to take to prevent transmission during pregnancy.

- **The baby needs to be delivered quickly.** An emergency C-section delivery can be necessary in fetal distress, in umbilical cord prolapse, in some cases of uterine bleeding, or, occasionally, if the mother is seriously ill.

C-sections aren't without risks

Because it involves surgery, a cesarean section creates some risks that usually are not present at vaginal births:

- **Injury.** Although major complications are not common, there can be injury to other internal organs, such as the bladder, the ureters (the tubes that come down from the kidneys), and the bowel. Excessive bleeding can occur, leading to anemia (low blood count) or even the need for blood transfusion. On very rare occasions, there is an injury to the fetus during the surgery.

- **Anesthetic complications.** Some women react adversely to the anesthesia used during a cesarean, especially general anesthesia. It's also possible for some stomach contents to get into the lungs while under general anesthesia. In most cases, it is safer to have an epidural or spinal if possible.

- **Unexpected prematurity.** For a scheduled cesarean without labor, it is important to be sure the baby is fully mature, especially if there is some uncertainty about the due date, or if the birth is planned before 38 completed weeks. If there is a reason to schedule a cesarean before labor begins, amniocentesis, in which a bit of amniotic fluid is drawn out of the uterus with a thin needle (see page 94), can help ensure that the baby's organs are mature enough to handle the outside world. This prevents accidentally timing the birth too early, leading to newborn respiratory problems or other complications of preterm birth.

Schedule a hospital or birth-center tour

As you get to the end of this month, it is time to do yourself a favor: Pack a bag for the hospital *before* you go into labor. Throwing things into a suitcase is not something you want to do when you're in the midst of strong contractions. While we're on that subject, you probably don't want to find your way to the hospital for the first time during labor, either. Many hospitals offer a tour, which includes information on routine procedures, where to park, what the labor-and-delivery rooms look like, and how to get in quickly if you are in a hurry or it's after hours. If you aren't going to take a tour, at least do one dry run.

Think ahead about what to take with you. To help, we've compiled a handy list of things you might want to remember. You may not end up using all these items, but it's better to have them with you during labor than

---

PACKING CHECKLIST FOR LABOR

☐ Insurance card or hospital registration papers

☐ Favorite pillow

☐ Special picture or object that makes you feel good (You can use it as a focal point as you breathe through contractions.)

☐ Bathrobe (Remember, those hospital gowns open in the back!)

☐ Slippers (for walking the halls as your labor progresses)

☐ Socks (It can get cold in bed.)

☐ Lollipops (to keep your mouth moist)

☐ Lip balm (The dry air in the hospital, as well as breathing exercises, can take a toll on your lips.)

☐ Toothbrush and toothpaste (You'd be surprised how refreshing it is to brush your teeth.)

---

to regret what you left at home. (However, it may be reassuring to know that if you turn up at the hospital empty handed, the staff always has extra necessities, such as toothbrushes and shampoo, available.)

☐ CD or tape player and your favorite relaxing music

☐ Lotion or oil (for a massage from your husband or labor coach)

☐ Tennis ball (to rub on your lower back as counterpressure)

☐ Barrette or hair band

☐ Eyeglasses (if you wear them—some hospitals don't allow contact lenses while in labor)

☐ Flash camera with extra rolls of film and extra batteries

☐ Video camera (if allowed)

☐ Phone list of friends and relatives

☐ Baby book (if you want to have footprints made)

In addition, don't forget about what you'll need after the baby is born. Consider gathering together a separate group of items you'll want to have with you

PACKING CHECKLIST FOR POSTPARTUM

☐ **Clothing.** Nightgowns or sweat suits are convenient and comfortable. You may want to wear a hospital gown the first 24 hours, however, because you may be bleeding significantly and won't want to risk staining your own clothes. Bring loose-fitting clothes to wear home.

☐ **Socks.** A few pairs of socks really can make a difference, since few maternity wards are carpeted.

☐ **Maternity or large-size underwear.** The underwear you wore while pregnant should serve you well. While your waist size will decrease dramatically after birth, don't expect to fit back into your pre-pregnancy underwear right away.

☐ **Bras.** Two or three comfortable nursing bras, or soft, exercise-type bras if you plan to bottle-feed your baby.

☐ **Toiletries.** These include shampoo, soap, toothbrush, toothpaste, lotion, deodorant, hairbrush, and any makeup.

after your baby has arrived. Some suggestions are listed below.

☐ **Extra-absorbent sanitary pads.** Many hospitals provide only the kind that require a belt, so bring ones that you'll find more comfortable.

☐ **Glasses.** Even if you normally wear contacts, you may have your hands full and not want to deal with the hassle of caring for them.

☐ **A calling card.** Most hospitals don't allow cell phones, since the signal can interfere with medical equipment. You'll be compelled to make your calls from a hospital phone, which can add up quickly. In the excitement to share your good news, you may not care, but you might feel differently when the hospital bill arrives. Buying a calling card in advance might save you a bundle.

☐ **Books or magazines.** Just in case you get a little down-time.

☐ **Baby clothes.** Consider packing an outfit that covers your infant's feet. At least bring socks: A newborn's hands and feet tend to get cold regardless of the temperature. And don't forget a baby hat.

☐ **Baby blanket.** You'll need one to wrap your baby in for the trip home.

☐ **Diapers.** Although the hospital nursery will undoubtedly supply them during your stay, it doesn't hurt to bring a few extras with you.

☐ **Car seat.** Whatever you do, don't forget this one! Hospitals these days won't let a baby leave without an

Now's the time to think about how to feed your newborn

You may already know how you plan to feed your baby, or you may have lots of questions and concerns about what will be best. While most parents have heard that breastfeeding provides the best nutrition and antibodies to help fight infection, many also have heard that bottle-feeding is easier or less stressful. In truth, both methods of feeding can result in wonderful, healthy babies, and the best choice is the one that works for you and your family. If you are on the fence, keep in mind that many families successfully combine breastfeeding and bottle-feeding to get the benefits of each. To learn more, be sure to check out the extensive infant car seat. It's a good idea to put it in the car before you go into labor, and have it checked by a car-safety professional to make sure that it's installed properly. You can find a free inspection facility near you by contacting the National Highway Traffic Safety Administration at www.nhtsa.gov.

sections on breastfeeding and formula-feeding in *Dr. Spock's Baby Basics* by Dr. Robert Needlman, another of the *Take Charge Parenting Guides*.

Q: I'm about to give birth to my first baby, and after reading about all the benefits of breastfeeding, I'm going to give it a try. Is there anything I should do ahead of time to help ensure a successful experience?

A: Yes, there are many things you can do to help prepare for breastfeeding. I always recommend reading about breastfeeding ahead of time, but you sound as if you've already done your "homework," which is great. The more you know about breastfeeding, the more confident you'll be, and the better able to handle any problems that might come up.

It's also a good idea to discuss your choice with your spouse or partner, the baby's grandparents and other close relatives, and the pediatrician you've chosen, to be sure you enlist their support. In addition, you might want to line up a lactation consultant for *expert advice. Your doctor, midwife, hospital, or childbirth-preparation-class teacher should be able to give you some referrals, or you can contact a breastfeeding support organization such as La Leche League. If you've already engaged a doula (see page 179), you may be all set: Her duties usually include helping you and the baby get started breastfeeding.*

You also might begin preparing your body for its new role. Women who have inverted or flat nipples sometimes have trouble breastfeeding; if you think this might be a problem in your case, speak with your doctor, midwife, or lactation specialist.

Finally, all moms-to-be who plan on nursing should be fitted with one or two nursing bras in the last month of pregnancy. Don't buy too many, though: Your breast size is likely to change once your milk comes in, and you may need a larger size.

NOTES

Use this space to jot down observations about your pregnancy or questions to ask your healthcare practitioner at your next visit:

_____

_____

_____

_____

_____

_____

_____

_____

_____

_____

_____

CHAPTER 9

Weeks 36—40

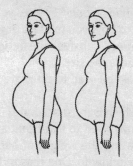

In these few last weeks of pregnancy, you may notice a change in your baby's position. Instead of riding high in your abdomen (as in the figure on the left), the baby drops deep into your pelvis (as in the figure on the right). The baby is said to have "engaged," bringing him one step closer to delivery.

ABOUT YOUR BABY

Get ready, world: Your baby is about to make her debut. All her organs and internal systems have formed, all her senses have developed. She is simply gaining weight and growing now, readying herself for life outside the warm, watery universe of the womb. At term, the average baby is 18 to 21 inches long and weighs a little more than 7 pounds. Of course, your baby may not be average, and weights from 5½ pounds to more than 9 pounds are common—and perfectly healthy.

There are three ways to estimate what a baby's size will be:

1. If you have had a baby before, you can compare how big you are to how you felt last time.
2. Your practitioner can feel the fetus through your abdomen and guess the size.
3. Ultrasound can be used to estimate the weight.

Can you guess which is most accurate?

You may be surprised to learn that a mother usually is best at estimating the weight of her fetus, followed by the doctor or midwife. One reason that feeling the abdomen isn't that accurate for estimating weight is that the practitioner is feeling your abdominal wall, your uterus, the baby, plus the liter (about four cups) of fluid that surrounds the fetus at term. While ultrasound seems most scientific, the formulas used to estimate the weight from measurements just aren't that accurate: They can be off by as much as 15 percent, which is more than a pound.

ABOUT YOU

As you reach the last few weeks of your pregnancy, you may notice that suddenly it is easier to breathe, and there seems to be more space between your breasts and your uterus. This change may occur over the course of a single day or more gradually, over a week or two. Your food may be a little easier to digest, and if you were suffering from heartburn, you may notice improvement.

"Engagement" comes early for first-time moms

This change probably signals that your baby has "dropped," as people often say—that is, he's engaged deep into your pelvis, positioning himself for labor. Engagement (also called "lightening," because your upper abdomen feels lighter) may occur for first-time moms days or even weeks before you actually give birth. For women who have had other children, engagement may not occur until labor is in progress.

While engagement is often welcomed as a tangible sign that birth is near, there is a downside: While your upper abdomen may be more comfortable, many women experience more pelvic pressure as the baby's head rests low in the pelvis. This increased pressure can make walking quite a challenge, and you may find yourself frequently hurrying to the bathroom, since there is now more pressure on your bladder.

Unfortunately, there isn't a lot you can do to make yourself more comfortable as this natural process takes place. To ease the pressure, you can try swimming, which will also help keep you active toward the end of pregnancy. Performing pelvic tilts (see page 168) or elevating your hips on a pillow may alleviate some of the discomfort as well. And just lying down will take the pressure off your pelvic bones for a while.

If this is your first child, engagement is evidence

that your baby should fit through the birth canal. First babies that have dropped are less likely to need to be born by cesarean than babies who are floating up out of the pelvis. Although you may be more uncomfortable now, remind yourself that it is normal for babies to drop toward the end of pregnancy. Even though childbirth may still be a few weeks away, you are one step closer to your ultimate goal.

You may not be able to see 'em, but you know your feet are swollen

Just when you think that pregnancy has wrought all the changes and surprises possible on your body, a new crop of symptoms is likely to turn up in this last month of pregnancy. One extremely common phenomenon is swelling, which can appear in the legs, hands, and feet.

During pregnancy, there is a normal increase in overall blood volume. For a variety of reasons, this increased fluid can escape out of the blood vessels and into the tissues. The resultant swelling is most commonly seen in the feet, since gravity pulls fluid down to them. Even if your feet don't look any different, you may still have a feeling of puffiness and your shoes may feel tight. Hot weather or eating a high-sodium meal can make it worse. In rare cases, swelling can be severe, making walking difficult.

Lying down or elevating your feet when sitting sometimes helps. The best treatment is swimming or any sort of total body immersion in cool water. The water pressure on the skin forces the tissue fluid back into the veins. In addition, although some salt is necessary in pregnancy, avoiding very salty or spicy foods may alleviate the problem a little. Water pills usually aren't recommended for swelling in pregnancy. Some women swear by support hose, while others think they just add to the uncomfortable feeling of pressure. The stockings come in both prescription and over-the-counter varieties, and in different strengths. If you opt for the pantyhose style, make sure that the stockings are designed for maternity use, so they aren't too tight across your expanding tummy.

The good news is that swelling resolves within a week or two after the baby is born. The fluid that has leaked into your tissues returns to the veins and is cleared from the body through your kidneys. If you had a cesarean or a lot of intravenous fluids during labor, it may take a few weeks for the fluid to be cleared and the swelling to improve. Keep in mind that if you had a lot of swelling, you can expect a lot of urine output.

Swelling in your hands can lead to carpal tunnel syndrome

If you begin to experience numbness or pain in your hands during the last few months of your pregnancy, you are not alone. Carpal tunnel syndrome usually affects the thumb, index finger, middle finger, and part of the ring finger of either or both hands. Generally, this condition can develop in people who have occupations that require repetitive use of the hands, such as typing, playing piano, or cutting meat, but in pregnancy

WHEN SWELLING IS A DANGER SIGN 🏍

Swelling that accumulates rapidly, extends to the face, or is accompanied by severe headache or high blood pressure can be a sign of preeclampsia, a serious condition that needs prompt medical attention (see page 231). If you are already being followed for high blood pressure, or if any of these other signs develop, call your practitioner.

almost anyone can get it. When the hand is bent back, such as when speaking on the telephone, the problem can be particularly annoying.

To understand carpal tunnel syndrome, you have to understand a little about the anatomy of your hands and arms. The nerves to the affected fingers run through a bony tunnel in the wrist. During pregnancy, this tunnel, like many other parts of the body, can become swollen. Pressure on the nerves caused by the swelling can cause numbness, tingling, burning, and pain in the affected fingers. Many pregnant women notice the symptoms during the night and first thing in the morning, when gravity allows the fluid that has accumulated in their legs during the day to redistribute to the rest of the body.

If you find that you experience symptoms of carpal tunnel syndrome during certain activities such as typing, try being careful about your positioning. An ergonomic keyboard, mouse, and keyboard pads, as well as a chair with adjustable arms, are some of the things that work wonders to relieve the strain on your arms and wrists. If the symptoms occur during telephone conversations, consider a speakerphone or headset.

If your symptoms are severe, you may want to discuss with your practitioner whether wearing a wrist brace is recommended. Most people with carpal tunnel syndrome experience at least some relief of symptoms by using a splint or brace to maintain the wrist in a neutral (slightly bent) position.

Typically, carpal tunnel symptoms will diminish after the birth of the baby, just as swelling in other parts of your body will resolve. If you continue to experience carpal tunnel symptoms after you give birth, tell your doctor.

PARENT TO PARENT

"I recently went to the doctor for swelling in my hands—couldn't get my rings off. She told me that this, in addition to the numbness/tingling sensation at night, is carpal tunnel syndrome. She said that if it gets worse, I might need to wear braces on my wrists, and that I should avoid sleeping on my hands."

—**HeatherT,** AS POSTED ON DRSPOCK.COM

Fatigue may be back again

Mid-pregnancy, most women find that their energy level is back to normal or even increased. But the last trimester of their pregnancies can be another story: Fatigue, which might have been your constant companion during the first trimester, may return with a vengeance.

There can be many causes. Between the parade of nocturnal trips to the bathroom and the nighttime discomforts of late pregnancy, moms-to-be often have difficulty sleeping. Some find that their minds are constantly in motion, thinking of things that need to be done to prepare for the new arrival. They also may be worried about the impending labor and delivery, or whether the baby will be healthy. Add to that the daytime work of carrying around extra weight and feeling swollen. Women who have had many children often feel more exhausted. Whether this is due to the accumulated wear and tear wrought by prior pregnancies or the demands of family responsibilities isn't clear—probably both.

What can you do to feel more rested?

- Eat healthful, nutritious meals.
- Exercise regularly to boost your energy level.
- Try to gain only a moderate amount of weight. The more weight you are carrying, the more tired you may be, and it's easy to pack on the pounds during this last stretch.
- Get enough sleep when possible, and listen to your body when it tells you that you need to rest.

- During the day, try to take short breaks and find a quiet place where you can put up your feet and close your eyes for a few minutes. If you are at work, you could rest during your lunch break, but make sure you leave time enough to eat.

- If you have other children, it can be hard to get a break in your day. Try to lie down at the same time your other children are napping. If they don't nap, try telling them it is quiet time and Mommy needs to rest.

Do what you can to get enough sleep, or at least rest. Taking care of yourself now will help keep you strong for the physical demands of labor and at your best for when your new baby comes home.

GETTING GOOD CARE

You may notice that your doctor or midwife has scheduled your prenatal visits more frequently at this point. While it is often helpful to have extra contact as labor gets closer, the real reason for the appointments is to screen for developing problems. The third trimester usually goes well, but there are some potential complications that we watch for extra closely around now, even in healthy, low-risk moms.

Preeclampsia can strike women without risk factors

For instance, did you ever wonder why your blood pressure is measured at every prenatal visit? And why your urine is checked for protein? Your practitioner is watching for a condition of pregnancy known as preeclampsia. It is also known as pregnancy-induced hypertension or by the older term *toxemia*.

Most expectant mothers experience a decrease in blood pressure in the second trimester. Later in the pregnancy, blood pressure usually returns to normal, but about seven percent of women will overshoot the mark and develop high blood pressure. A blood pressure of 140/90 or above is typically considered to be elevated. Some women have blood pressures in that range even when not pregnant; for them, a "high" blood pressure during pregnancy may be less of a concern, since they always run high. On the other hand, if a woman's blood pressure usually runs low, a rise in blood pressure during pregnancy (even if the pressure stays below 140/90) might still be considered elevated.

In most cases, a slightly elevated blood pressure causes no harm to mother or baby. However, if mildly elevated blood pressure is accompanied by protein in the urine, swelling in the hands and face, or changes in certain blood tests, the diagnosis is preeclampsia.

The symptoms of preeclampsia are different for each patient, and many also can occur in normal pregnancies, such as:

- swelling in the face, hands, or feet
- sudden weight gain (such as five pounds in one week)
- persistent severe headache

- constant spots before the eyes
- pain in the upper abdomen.

Women who experience any of these symptoms should call their doctor or practitioner right away. They may need to see a healthcare professional to make sure that they are not developing preeclampsia.

In rare, severe cases, preeclampsia can cause the mother to have temporary liver or kidney dysfunction or even seizures (eclampsia). Very high blood pressures can lead to a stroke. This severe level of hypertension is quite rare in pregnant women who have not had blood-pressure problems before pregnancy.

Many women who get preeclampsia have no risk factors other than the fact that they are in their first full-term pregnancy. There is also an increased likelihood of preeclampsia in women who already have high blood pressure (or had hypertension in a previous pregnancy), or are carrying twins or triplets, are over 40 or less than 16 years of age, are diabetic, or are very overweight.

Nothing has been shown to prevent preeclampsia in first-time, low-risk mothers. Some prevention strategies for higher-risk patients have been proposed, but none has been found to be reliable. Seizures usually can be prevented by treatment with an intravenous infusion of magnesium sulfate during labor and for 24 hours after childbirth.

Preeclampsia is a temporary condition that resolves promptly after delivery. Sometimes induction of labor, or even a cesarean, is needed to speed delivery if the mother is getting sick. After the baby is born, the mother's symptoms start to resolve within minutes to hours in most cases. Blood pressure may take a few weeks to return to normal, but usually is out of the danger zone before the mother and baby leave the hospital.

If preeclampsia is diagnosed and your baby is not near his due date, you may be instructed to rest as much as possible on your left side and return for office visits more frequently. In rare cases, preeclampsia may become severe enough that delivery of a premature baby is the only option. While this is a serious step to take, it is done only when a mother's health is at stake (and therefore her baby's health as well).

Remember: Most mothers with preeclampsia have healthy babies and are back to their usual state of good health soon after childbirth.

Bleeding is not uncommon in late pregnancy

If you find spots of blood on your underwear or toilet paper, it's sure to prove worrisome to you, but there's no need to panic. Keep in mind that, most of the time, the cause is never discovered and the bleeding usually stops on its own and poses no real danger. It's also important to note that not all blood found on toilet paper is from the vagina. It's extremely common to experience bleeding from the rectum during pregnancy. Most of the time it comes from small tears in the rectal lining caused by constipation. Sometimes hemorrhoids bleed, and you may occasionally have blood in your urine because of a bladder infection.

If the vagina is definitely the source of the bleeding, there can be several causes, some serious, others not. Bleeding from the cervix is not uncommon after intercourse, a pelvic exam, or a Pap smear. Some light bleeding at the end of pregnancy, near the due date, can be normal. Pink, greenish, or brown mucus discharge, as I've mentioned earlier, is sometimes called bloody show, and can signal cervical dilation and passage of the mucus plug.

It's important to remember that bleeding before the ninth month, or any bleeding that goes beyond just spotting, should be reported to your practitioner. Heavy or brisk bleeding of bright red blood that fills up a sanitary pad, or the passing of clots, needs to be reported to your doctor promptly. This type of bleeding might indicate a potentially serious condition of pregnancy:

- **Placenta previa.** This problem occurs when the placenta is located low in the uterus, covering the internal opening of the cervix. Placenta previa usually can be seen by ultrasound. If the placenta is disturbed by contractions, intercourse, or pelvic examination, it can start to bleed. Keep in mind that this is the mother's blood, not the baby's. Usually the bleeding will stop on its own, but it can be quite heavy. Depending on the exact situation—the maturity of the baby and the degree of the bleeding—a decision may be made for delivery by cesarean section. It is important to know that while placenta previa is often seen on ultrasound early in the pregnancy, it frequently moves out of the way by the third trimester and doesn't cause any problems.

- **Placental abruption.** In placental abruption, the placenta becomes dislodged from the wall of the uterus, allowing the mother's blood to collect behind it and eventually make its way to the vagina. This collection of blood often irritates the uterus, causing contractions. Surprisingly, the baby can remain healthy using only the part of the placenta that is still attached. If the detachment continues, certain warning signs that your doctor will screen for might necessitate delivery, even if the baby isn't yet full-term.

BLEEDING IN RH-NEGATIVE MOTHERS

Mothers with Rh-negative blood (see page 149) who may be carrying an Rh-positive fetus should get an Rh immunoglobulin (RhoGam) shot whenever there is the chance that significant mixing of fetal blood into the mother's circulation has occurred. This may happen if any significant vaginal bleeding takes place in pregnancy.

If problems occur, your doctor will check how the baby is doing

If you start to develop preeclampsia, bleeding, or other problems during late pregnancy and your health is stable, your practitioner will take steps to watch your baby extra closely to be sure he is tolerating the situation. If signs of distress develop, labor can be induced or a cesarean can be performed, depending on the situation. As discussed earlier, a baby who is moving regularly demonstrates that she is in good condition (see page 205). Another method of assessing fetal well-being is a type of monitoring known as nonstress testing.

Nonstress testing measures the fetal heart rate

Nonstress testing (NST) involves monitoring a developing baby's resting heart rate without inducing contractions, as we do in a contraction stress test (see page 263). The fetal monitor has two belts that go around the mother's waist. One sensor registers any contractions that may occur (sometimes they're so subtle, the mother doesn't notice them); the other tracks the fetal heart rate. These are graphed on paper or on a computer screen, and you often can see the graph as it is being made. Usually, the NST is not uncomfortable, although it may get tiresome to stay in one position for 20 minutes or so. (In fact, it's not unusual for these tests to run as long as an hour.)

The usual fetal heart rate is between 120 and 160 beats per minute. This is called the baseline rate. Once the monitor is in place, your practitioner will look for certain measurements to see how the baby is faring, including if his heart rate rises above his baseline when he moves. An NST is considered reassuring if there are at least two accelerations of the fetal heart rate of at least 15 beats per minute, lasting at least 15 seconds, occurring within a 20-minute time block. This is called a reactive NST. If these accelerations don't occur, the test is said to be nonreactive. In addition, since many women have mild contractions that they may not even notice, your practitioner will note any of the baby's responses to contractions or if the fetal heart rate dips below the baseline.

A fetus who is sleeping may not show any accelerations. You and your practitioner will have to wait for him to wake up, or sometimes you can wake him with stimulation. Although a reactive NST is a good sign, a nonreactive NST does not mean the baby is in trouble. If you and your practitioner aren't reassured by the results of the NST, more testing is usually done. This might include a more prolonged NST, a contraction stress test, or a biophysical profile (see page 265).

LOOKING AHEAD

With your due date approaching, you're probably thinking more and more about what labor and delivery will be like, especially if you're a first-time mom. To help you get prepared, I'll go into a little more detail about some of the events of childbirth in this section, and give you plenty of information about both medical and natural ways to deal with pain.

Breaking your water is sometimes the first sign of labor

It's a scene that's been played for drama or comic relief in countless movies and TV shows: An unsuspecting pregnant woman's water breaks—usually at the least convenient time possible—causing a great rush of water, and her flustered husband whisks her away to the hospital. In actuality, however, the breaking of water (really amniotic fluid) isn't necessarily the opening bell signaling labor and delivery.

Amniotic fluid is clear, with an odor that has been compared to a scouring cleanser. The fluid is held inside the uterus by a sac made of thin, translucent membranes. When a hole develops in the membranes, the fluid is released. This is what is referred to as breaking your water. The water can break before or after labor starts.

When your water breaks, you may notice a popping sensation and either a gush or a trickle as some of the amniotic fluid leaks out through your vagina (it may even run down your leg). Some mothers-to-be are not sure what is happening: *Did the baby just kick my bladder or did my bag of water break?* (One mom told me that she'd been sleeping in a waterbed and was convinced that the bed had sprung a leak!)

If it is a big gush, it may be obvious that your water has broken. If there is just a trickle, you'll want to put on a sanitary pad and lie down for 30 minutes or so. If you feel a small gush when you get up, even though you don't feel any contractions or other labor symptoms, it's possible that your amniotic sac has indeed ruptured, and you should notify your practitioner.

A nurse or doctor can do a test in the office if it isn't clear whether or not your water has broken. This feels a bit like a Pap test. Using a speculum to see inside your vagina, your practitioner will take a sample of the fluid with a cotton-tipped applicator and test the pH. She also may put some on a glass slide and examine it under the microscope. Sometimes these tests don't clearly show that the membranes have broken, because fluid can leak intermittently and might not leak during your exam. Ultrasound may be helpful to see how much fluid remains around the baby, although the quantity can vary for a number of reasons.

If you are close to your due date and have ruptured your membranes, labor usually begins within 24 hours. If your water breaks at term and labor has not yet begun, many practitioners recommend inducing labor in order to prevent infection from entering the uterus, now that the protective sac has a hole in it.

Once your water breaks, the fluid may continue to leak until you deliver your baby. This happens because amniotic fluid is still being produced, and pockets of fluid usually remain around the baby. Some mothers worry about a "dry birth" if they break their water before labor, but there is no such thing!

Telling real labor from false alarms

As I discussed in Chapter 6, your uterus begins to contract in your third trimester, sometimes as early as the end of your second. You may not notice the sensation, or it may feel like a tightening or a low, menstrual-like cramp. The baby may seem to be balling up. This, of course, is not the baby, but the uterine muscle tightening. These early contractions are called Braxton-Hicks contractions (see page 141), named after the obstetrician who first described them. Even Braxton-Hicks contractions can sometimes be painful, making it hard to tell true labor from false.

To complicate things further, false-labor contractions may even come at regular five-minute intervals, lasting about 30 seconds. This may go on for hours. Even women who already have had children go to the hospital thinking they are in real labor and find out it was a false alarm.

True vs. false labor

Here are a few guidelines to help you distinguish true from false labor:

	False labor	True labor
Timing of contractions	Often irregular; not usually becoming closer together.	Contractions come regularly, usually four to six minutes apart, and can become closer together. Usually last 30 to 70 seconds.
Strength of contractions	Frequently weak, not getting stronger with time. Or a strong contraction is followed by weaker ones.	Become stronger with time. You also may feel vaginal pressure.
Pain with contractions	Usually felt in the front only.	Can start in the back and move to the front.
Position changes and hydration	Contractions may stop or slow down when you walk, lie down, change position, or increase your fluid intake.	Contractions continue no matter what position changes you make or how much you drink.

Should you stay or should you go?

If this is a first pregnancy, you are much more likely to go to your hospital or birth center too early rather than too late. Once you are past 36 weeks, I usually recommend ignoring contractions until they are very strong and regular. (Before that time, it is best to call your practitioner if you have any concerns about labor, since preterm labor is easier to stop if it hasn't advanced too far.) At term, if you think labor may be starting, try taking a nap or a walk, rather than focusing on timing your contractions. Many first-time moms exhaust themselves tracking contractions before they are even in active labor. Generally, you don't have to time them until you can't hold a conversation during one and have to focus on relaxing. Often, by that point, they may be two or three minutes apart. Expect to go to the hospital when the contractions are quite strong, closer than four or five minutes apart, and continue in that pattern for over an hour.

For women who have given birth before, I usually recommend using your previous labor as a guideline. On average, second babies come in half the time it took for the first. Subsequent pregnancies are usually similar to the second one. Keep in mind that these are just general guidelines. Talk to your practitioner about specific recommendations for your individual situation.

If you just aren't sure whether it is false or real labor, don't feel bad going in to be examined. Your practitioner and the nurses there see many women each day in false labor. Sometimes it is hard even for the professionals to tell if it's the real thing.

You can prepare yourself to deal with the pain of labor

As your due date draws closer, you're sure to be thinking about the pain of labor—in particular, what the pain will be like and how you will handle it. Certainly, every woman's experience is different, and pain perception varies by individual, but it's safe to say that most women feel some discomfort during labor.

If this is your first time going through childbirth, it will be difficult for you to imagine what labor will feel like. Some women describe contractions as feeling like severe intestinal cramps. Others feel most of the pressure in their backs and hardly notice the tightening in the front. By active labor, you generally can't hold a normal conversation during a contraction—you are busy getting through it. In some ways, labor is like running a long-distance race: There may come a time that you feel you can't go on, but the encouragement of those around you can help you find inner strength.

You can best prepare for the experience of labor by becoming familiar with the normal process of labor and with all your options, from nonmedical comfort measures to high-tech anesthesia. Be sure to discuss pain relief with your healthcare provider in advance so that you know what will be available when your baby's birthday arrives.

Natural pain-relief methods can offer comfort during labor

If you choose to go the nonmedical route, a great number of activities can ease your discomfort. Many women have found the following techniques to be useful alternatives (or additions) to medication:

- **Water therapy.** Indulge in a warm shower or bath; it can be both calming and relaxing. If you are feeling labor pains in your back, water massage can be particularly helpful. Some birth centers and hospitals are set up for water births, where you actually have your baby in the tub (see page 21).

- **Distraction.** Sometimes, particularly in early labor, doing some sort of activity can take your mind off

---

Q: Why is there pain when you have a baby?

A: This is a great question. It really made me think! While some mothers say their labors weren't really painful, most agree with your perception that there is some pain involved. Why would this be? I'm not sure anyone knows the entire answer, but here are four factors that may play a role:

- In humans, evolution had to find a balance between head size (and the importance of having a big brain) and the size and shape of the pelvic bones (so that the female could still walk and run). Because of this delicate balance, it is a tighter fit for humans to give birth than for most other animals. The mother's body has to work very hard to maneuver the baby through the birth canal.

- The cervix, which is the opening to the uterus, sends pain signals to the brain as it is being stretched open. During labor it has to open 10 impending contractions. Instead of waiting for the next pain to come, watch TV, read, play cards, go for a walk, or call a friend. Music can totally change the mood in a hospital room; consider packing a portable stereo and some relaxing tapes or CDs in your baby bag.

centimeters (about four inches) to allow the baby's head to fit through.

- During contractions, the muscle of the uterus doesn't get a lot of oxygen, and lack of oxygen to any tissue can cause pain.
- The opening of the vagina also has to stretch to allow the baby's head to pass through. This occurs as the baby is being born, and can be painful.

There are lots of factors, though, that affect our perception of pain. Fear makes us feel pain more strongly. Distraction and relaxation tend to minimize pain. And, of course, pain medications can greatly diminish the sensation of discomfort. So while nearly all women say that their labors were painful, most do find them manageable, and are even willing to do it again in order to bring another baby into the world.

- **Breathing and relaxation.** You'll learn about different breathing techniques in your childbirth education classes. These exercises serve partly as
  distraction and partly as a way to calm yourself.
  They also remind you not to hold your breath during pain. A deep-relaxation technique called hypnotherapy has been immensely helpful for some
  mothers-to-be. Classes in hypnotherapy, sometimes called self-hypnosis, are available in many
  communities.

- **Effleurage.** This is a method of lightly massaging
  your abdomen (which can be done by you or your
  coach) as you have a contraction. Using both hands,
  start at your pubic bone and stroke lightly up and
  out to your sides. Then gently slide your hands
  toward the center of your abdomen and down to
  the pubic bone. Make circular motions with each
  hand on either side of your abdomen.

- **Massage.** Light touch may feel wonderful on certain parts of your body, but you may prefer the
  added pressure of a deeper massage on other
  areas. Your coach can note where your body is
  tense and work on that area as a reminder to stay
  relaxed.

- **Acupressure and acupuncture.** These age-old techniques were developed in China for treatment
  of many medical conditions, including pain. Applying firm pressure (acupressure) or inserting and
  maneuvering fine needles (acupuncture) at certain
  areas of the body can be an effective form of pain

management. In some communities in the United States, licensed acupuncturists offer treatment during labor. For more information on acupuncture, visit the website for the National Center for Complementary and Alternative Medicine (NCCAM) at *http://nccam.nih.gov/*.

Medications can provide highly effective pain relief

Various medical options are available for each stage of labor. While most can be used throughout the birth process, some are best for early labor, some provide relief only during the delivery, and others are solely for cesarean sections. Your options include:

- **Systemic analgesia.** Narcotic medications, such as Demerol, morphine, and Nubain, are generally administered through an IV (intravenously), but occasionally they're given as a shot in the buttock. Narcotics take the edge off contractions so that, while you may still feel some pain, you won't care about it as much. They often cause drowsiness and may help you to get some rest. These medications also can cause nausea and may make some people feel confused or out of it. Sometimes, starting with a small test dose can allow you to be sure you feel OK on the medication before taking the whole amount.

  Although narcotics do cross the placenta, your metabolism removes the medication from the baby's system before birth, so no harm is done if they are given early or in the middle of labor. Systemic medications generally are not given close to the time of delivery, because being born with medication still in her system poses dangers to the baby, such as shallow breathing and slowed reflexes. If a baby does happen to be born with narcotics in her system, however, there are other medications that can be used to reverse these effects.

- **Spinal block.** A spinal block (also called a saddle block) is similar to an epidural in that a small amount of medication is injected into the fluid around your spinal cord. It completely numbs the lower half of your body for about 90 minutes, thus preventing pushing of any kind. A spinal is given for C-sections and sometimes for forceps deliveries.

- **Pudendal block.** The anesthetic—a numbing medication such as lidocaine—is injected through the wall of the vagina into the pudendal nerve on each side to relieve pain at the vaginal opening as the baby comes out. It works fairly well and is extremely safe.

- **Local anesthesia.** A numbing medication (most commonly lidocaine) is injected directly into the area between the vagina and the rectum just before an episiotomy (see page 288) is performed or before the baby is born. Most practitioners also will use local anesthesia when repairing a tear in the birth canal.

- **General anesthesia.** General anesthesia, also called going to sleep, usually is reserved for emergencies:

The baby needs to be delivered immediately by cesarean, with no time to place an epidural or spinal block. In rare cases where the mother cannot undergo an epidural or spinal for medical reasons, it's the only option.

General anesthesia typically is used only for cesarean births. You may receive oxygen by mask before the anesthesiologist administers the medication through an IV. Sleep comes within seconds, so you'll feel no pain. Doctors will insert a tube into your throat to help you breathe during surgery. Because general anesthetics cross the placenta, the baby is delivered quickly once you're asleep.

Epidurals are often a mom's first choice

I've saved what many women consider the best medicated pain-relief option for last: epidural anesthesia. It's used to relieve pain in childbirth more often than any other anesthetic. While some hospitals don't have epidural anesthesia available, the rate of epidural use during births can be as much as 80 percent at some institutions.

An epidural works by distributing small amounts of medication into the nerves around the spinal cord through a thin catheter in your back. It relieves the pain of your contractions but still allows you to feel touch. You may experience some numbness in your legs, but you'll probably be able to move them. In most cases, you must remain in bed when you have an epidural because of the loss of feeling in your legs.

Some hospitals now offer "walking epidurals," which help with discomfort but don't make your legs feel weak.

Because an epidural numbs the birth canal, it also may lessen pain from pushing as the baby descends during delivery. Although the pushing stage may last longer with an epidural, most women still feel the urge to push and are able to do so quite effectively. We have learned from recent research that if a mother with an epidural doesn't start pushing until the baby descends and she feels the urge, she's more efficient at pushing and is less likely to get exhausted before the baby has arrived. This means that she doesn't start to push just because she is completely dilated; instead, the team waits patiently until the baby has descended farther and the mother feels more pressure in the vagina. In some cases where the mother gets exhausted from pushing too long, or if her urge to push isn't strong, the baby may have to be helped out with vacuum or forceps (see page 290).

In addition to providing excellent pain relief for labor with minimal risk to the mother or baby, an epidural is sometimes recommended for medical reasons. This is common in the case of twins, or if cesarean delivery is likely. Sometimes the relaxation that a woman can get with pain relief can help labor to progress, and if she is holding back from pushing because of pain, she may actually push better with an epidural in place. Your practitioner may suggest an epidural as a strategy if labor is not progressing well.

HOW AN EPIDURAL IS PLACED 🐾

If you opt for an epidural, you may be seated at the edge of your bed or lying on your side. The middle of your back is washed with a disinfecting solution. A surgical drape may cover most of your back. After the practitioner feels your back to find the best spot, an injection of numbing medicine is given.

As a second, firmer needle goes in, many women feel pressure or a twinge. A small plastic tube (catheter) is slipped through the needle, and the needle is withdrawn. The catheter resembles the intravenous catheter that is used for IVs. The epidural catheter remains near, but not in, your spinal cord.

Pain medicine is dripped through the epidural catheter onto the nerves as they emerge from the spinal cord. As labor continues, the amount of the medicine can be adjusted to obtain the right level of pain relief.

An epidural is the most common anesthetic for cesarean deliveries as well, because pain relief is excellent and the medication doesn't harm the baby. With increased dosage of the anesthetic given through the epidural catheter, you can become totally numb from the abdomen down. Sometimes women having cesareans feel touch or a pushing sensation, but there should be no pain. After surgery, many hospitals administer a long-lasting narcotic or leave the epidural catheter in place to provide pain relief without drowsiness; lower doses are given so that you regain normal strength and sensation in your legs and can walk around.

PARENT TO PARENT

"I had two wonderful natural childbirths, both at birth centers using certified nurse-midwives. Midwives (and really progressive OBs) allow women to eat, drink, move around, walk, get into the tub, and do all the other things that help us be comfortable and speed up labor. When we are allowed to follow our instincts, labor is not unbearable, and birth can be such an empowering experience."

—**dwoconnor,** AS POSTED ON DRSPOCK.COM

"I had two deliveries in which I required epidurals, and here's how I see it: If you want to suffer the raw pain of delivery for some obscure reason, go for it. But I

Epidurals can have side effects

The vast majority of epidurals are placed and function without problems. Sometimes, however, they can cause muscle weakness, or patchy or one-sided pain relief.

One common side effect is that, after the epidural is placed, contractions seem to slow down. This may be due to the extra intravenous fluid given just before epidural placement. The contractions may come back

---

knew that I was going to give birth only a few times in my life and I wanted to enjoy them.

"The hardest part of an epidural is having to stay extremely still when the anesthesiologist administers it. Your initial feeling will be a very cold yet completely tolerable sensation down your back, and then your legs will have a delightful hum to them. You will be 'frozen' from pain in the mid section, where all the contractions are taking place. There's no screaming, no anger, no added stress. You'll be able to watch your babies being born in as comfortable a way as possible."

—**3boysmom**, AS POSTED ON DRSPOCK.COM

on their own, or Pitocin may be needed to restore their regularity.

Another undesired effect after epidural placement is the temporary slowing of some babies' heart rates. This may be related to a temporary drop in the mothers' blood pressure, and both usually resolve in a few moments with more IV fluid.

In very rare instances, the pain medication can end up where it is not intended. Medication can stray into the spinal fluid rather than staying just outside it, toward the top part of the body rather than to the lower part, or into the bloodstream. The anesthesiologist watches for these complications and treats any problems that develop.

The next day, a small percentage of women experience a specific kind of epidural-related headache (called spinal headache). This can be treated with rest, caffeine, or a procedure similar to epidural placement, called an epidural blood patch.

As I've said before, my best advice about pain relief is to set things up ahead of time to support your goals, but to realize that it's OK to change your mind as labor progresses. Childbirth is unpredictable, even for women who have had babies before. And remember: While the type of pain relief you use may seem like a pressing topic right now, the whole issue fades away as you behold your beautiful baby for the first time.

NOTES

Use this space to jot down observations about your pregnancy or questions to ask your healthcare practitioner at your next visit:

_____

_____

_____

_____

_____

_____

_____

_____

_____

_____

_____

_____

CHAPTER 10

Beyond Week 40

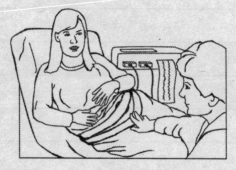

External fetal monitors give your practitioner valuable information about your baby's condition, which can be especially important if you go a week or so past your due date. These devices have two elastic straps that go around your abdomen. The electronic sensor under one strap records any contractions you might experience, while the sensor in the other measures your baby's heart rate. The feedback from the sensors is charted on a graph produced by the monitor.

ABOUT YOUR BABY

Some women tell their friends that they are 10 months' pregnant as a joke, but for some moms-to-be, it's actually true. As I mentioned in the beginning of this book, babies are no respecters of due dates. Your baby might fall into the 5 percent of newborns who "decide" to arrive right on time, but the vast majority come a little bit sooner or later. If your baby makes his entrance into this world a week or so before he is due, his arrival probably will come as a welcome surprise. But if you're in the roughly 33 percent of women whose babies come after their due dates, every passing day may make you more anxious and impatient. Since so many moms-to-be fall into this category, I'll explain what doctors call "post-dates" issues in this chapter, before we tackle some more events of birth in the next.

ABOUT YOU

I have to admit that dealing with late-coming newborns is an issue near and dear to my heart. When I was pregnant with my son, I went about a week (well, actually, eight whole days) past my due date. Of all people, I should have known not to get that one red-letter day too firmly set in my mind. And yet, hearing that date repeated at each prenatal visit, it was embedded in my brain: *July 15, July 15, July 15.* Maybe this isn't true for you. Maybe you understand, in your heart as well as in your mind, that due dates indicate a four-week period in which your baby is likely to arrive, not a specific day. And if you move into a post-date period, a much more useful mantra would be: *All babies come out, pregnancy won't last forever, there really will be a baby.* But even as you try to be patient, knowing that, in most cases, it's best for the baby to arrive on his own schedule, you might start wondering: *When is it safe to try to naturally induce labor, and how do I go about accomplishing that?*

Natural methods of inducing your own labor

If you go past your due date, you're sure to hear about all sorts of homegrown, natural methods of inducing labor. I'll run through the most popular here, but keep in mind that some of these are safer and more advisable than others. Also, remember that you shouldn't even consider trying *any* of them until you are around 40 weeks' pregnant or overdue. That's because your due date could be inaccurate, and if you start your labor before 40 weeks, you might give birth to the baby before he is ready to thrive outside the womb.

Use caution when trying any of these natural methods to begin your labor, particularly herbs and nipple stimulation. The uterus can become hyperstimulated, meaning that it'll get too little rest between contractions. This can cause the baby to receive less oxygen, resulting in fetal distress. That's one of the reasons why, before trying any of these techniques, it's very important to discuss the following with your practitioner:

- **Walking.** If you are having contractions but are not yet in labor, walking sometimes gets the ball rolling. Walking allows your hips to sway side to side, which will help bring the baby into position to be born. Also, by standing upright, you're using gravity to move the baby down into the pelvis. Another plus: It usually feels good to walk when you are having contractions. And, of course, even if you don't go into full-blown labor, at least you're getting some exercise.

- **Sex.** Making love can be one of the last things on a woman's mind toward the end of her pregnancy. Often she feels clumsy and big and may be experiencing a lot of vaginal pressure. But here's one fact that may put you in the mood: When you and your partner make love, his semen (which contains hormonelike substances called prostaglandins that influence metabolism and help ready your body for labor) can stimulate contractions. A double dose—a few hours apart—may give you even better results, though there haven't been any scientific studies to back up this claim.

- **Castor oil.** For decades, women have been drinking castor oil to help induce labor. In fact, many old-school physicians swear by it. It is believed to work by causing spasms in the intestines, which surround the uterus toward the end of pregnancy. These spasms, in turn, cause the uterus to cramp, which may result in starting labor or making your contractions stronger if you're already in early labor.

  You can take one to four ounces of castor oil, mixed with six ounces of orange juice to cut its oiliness. You'll want to drink it quickly because of the unpleasant taste. Some practitioners suggest taking a single dose; others suggest repeated doses,

depending on your response. Keep in mind that castor oil usually will cause your bowels to empty
within about three hours. With luck, soon after that
you will be in true labor.

- **Spicy food.** Some mothers swear that it was that
  extra-hot enchilada from their favorite Mexican
  restaurant that persuaded their babies it was time to
  come out. Unfortunately, the verdict is mixed on this
  one. You could try it, but if you have a full stomach
  when you are in labor, you might vomit and see that
  enchilada again—and under less-than-appetizing circumstances.

- **Blue and black cohosh.** These plants are often recommended by herbalists to induce labor. They may be
  particularly helpful if you are having weak or irregular
  contractions. Blue cohosh is believed to make uterine
  contractions stronger, while black cohosh may regu-
  late them. Together, they are supposed to make contractions more effective. Unfortunately, no studies
  have determined that this treatment is safe, or
  whether all versions of the herbs available for pur-
  chase are of equal potency. (Once again, be sure to
  discuss any herbal treatment with your practitioner to
  see if it is a good idea in your situation.)

- **Nipple stimulation.** Some women massage their
  nipples as a way to induce labor. This stimulation
  brings about the release of oxytocin, a natural form
  of Pitocin (see page 268). Oxytocin causes contractions, which sometimes evolve into labor. Most practitioners are not enthusiastic about this method
  because it can cause excessively long, strong uterine

contractions that can result in fetal distress. Unless your practitioner advises it and is monitoring your progress closely, nipple stimulation is *not* recommended as a means for beginning labor.

- **Stripping the membranes.** (Even though your practitioner would be the one to do this procedure, I include it here because it is a nonmedical intervention.) Your practitioner may offer to "strip your membranes" to help start your labor. This procedure usually feels like a vaginal examination, although it sometimes can be painful or cause cramping. The practitioner inserts her gloved finger through the cervix and sweeps the amniotic membranes free of their attachment to the lower part of the uterine cavity. This process is believed to release prostaglandins, which help thin out and dilate the cervix.

While some experts believe that stripping the membranes causes you to go into labor that day, the only published research on this procedure was done by a group of midwives who stripped the membranes of some of their patients at every visit to the office after 38 weeks' gestation. Their findings showed that patients who had their membranes stripped were less likely to go past their due dates. According to the study, the procedure didn't seem to pose any complications and didn't cause the mothers' waters to break.

So, just how successful are these natural methods? Frankly, if your body isn't prepared to go into labor, you can try them as much as your heart desires, but you will only frustrate yourself. It isn't even clear that any of these natural techniques are truly effective. Since everyone will go into labor eventually, some methods' good reputations may stem from reports of happy women who thought they were successful, when in reality the women were about to go into labor anyway. If it is necessary to induce labor for medical reasons, your practitioner will probably recommend a more conventional, in-hospital induction method (see page 268).

PARENT TO PARENT

"Just gave birth to a beautiful baby girl! If I had waited on Mother Nature, I'm convinced I'd STILL be pregnant—at 40 weeks, my body wasn't ready for delivery. My husband and I went into the hospital late Sunday night to prepare my unripe cervix for induction, and by Monday afternoon—after the breaking of my water, an epidural, and a Pitocin drip—we had our little girl. The placenta, however, took forever to come, but, honestly, by that time, I was too much in love with our baby to care."

—mrs. jewelmaker, AS POSTED ON DRSPOCK.COM

GETTING GOOD CARE

After the 40th week of pregnancy, there are some reasons to watch babies a little extra closely. Starting about a week after the due date, and earlier in some situations, practitioners want to be reassured that the baby has not outgrown her placenta. While the placenta stops growing at about 37 weeks, the baby keeps growing and needs the nutrients and oxygen that the placenta provides. While most babies manage quite well during this time, some babies show signs that the placenta is not supplying their needs as well as could be hoped, and would be better off cared for outside the womb.

As you get more than a week past your due date, you will be scheduled for frequent prenatal visits, and routine monitoring with nonstress testing (see page 237), contraction stress testing, or ultrasound. Since babies who move around regularly are showing that they are in good condition, you can keep track of your baby's movements to assure fetal well-being as the due date comes and goes (see page 205). A decrease in the normal pattern of your baby's activity should lead you to call your practitioner that day. In this case, you will be asked to come into the office or hospital so that the baby can be monitored with a nonstress test, contraction stress test, or biophysical profile to be sure everything is OK.

Contraction stress testing monitors how the baby's handling labor

Like the NST (see page 237), contraction stress testing, or CST, uses the fetal monitor to watch the baby's heart-rate pattern and to see how he handles the mild stress of contractions. The test is said to be adequate if there are three contractions in 10 minutes and the baby's heart rate doesn't go down in response. If you are having some contractions on your own, a scheduled nonstress test may meet these criteria and be counted as a contraction stress test. If you aren't having contractions, mild contractions can be induced with a short course of Pitocin (see page 268) or by having you stimulate your nipples. Even though nipple stimulation sounds like a nice, natural way to bring on contractions for this test, as I noted earlier, many practitioners have found that nipple-stimulation contractions sometimes come too quickly and last many minutes, creating enough stress to slow even a healthy baby's heart rate. If nipple stimulation is used to start contractions, it should be done with careful monitoring of the fetal heart and slowly increased stimuli, such as starting with just a warm washcloth on the breast. *Do not try this test at home.*

Usually the contractions of a CST are mild and the mother does not experience significant pain. As soon as contractions appear closer together than three in 10 minutes, the test is complete and the Pitocin or nipple stimulation is discontinued. If the baby's heart rate stays normal through the contractions, the CST is said to be negative, meaning that the baby is in good condition. Having a contraction stress test generally doesn't put you into labor.

Even though a contraction stress test may be positive (abnormal), as when the baby's heart rate slows down in response to contractions, the baby still has a good chance of being fine at birth. Many such babies even get all the way through labor without further problems. About half of the babies with a positive contraction stress test, however, will not be able to tolerate the contractions of labor and will need to be delivered by cesarean.

A biophysical profile helps assess your baby's condition

Another way of monitoring how your baby is doing is with a biophysical profile (BPP). This is a fancy name for a prolonged ultrasound, sometimes lasting more than half an hour, to monitor the baby's movements, body tone, and breathing efforts, as well as measure the volume of the amniotic fluid. Each of these four parameters is given a score of either zero or two points, then totaled up. A high score (8–10) means that the baby seems to be in good condition, while a low score (0–4) indicates that he might be better off outside the uterine environment. A score of 6 usually requires a repeat test within 12 to 24 hours.

Sometimes a modified BPP is done, which includes only a nonstress test and an ultrasound to check amniotic fluid volume. If both are normal, some experts find it as reassuring as a full BPP, which is a lot more time-consuming. Your practitioner will recommend which test—or set of tests—is worthwhile in your case.

Induction can be the best course of action under certain circumstances

If fetal testing indicates that the baby may be stressed, your practitioner probably will recommend prompt induction of labor. If your pregnancy is going fine and the baby's tests are reassuring, he may wait until one to two weeks after your due date before inducing. Once you reach two weeks after the due date, the chance of fetal stress in labor increases, and most doctors believe that a baby is better off in the nursery than in the womb. The dilation of the cervix, the confidence that the due date is correct, and the size of the baby may influence your practitioner's recommendations regarding induction.

Some parents-to-be want induction of labor as soon as they pass the due date. They may be frustrated about the wait or worried that the baby is growing too big to be delivered vaginally. But it usually is better to let nature take its course. It turns out that for first-time mothers, inducing labor results in more cesarean sections (because the cervix doesn't open) than just waiting for labor to start on its own. Even a big baby has a good chance of being delivered vaginally if he tucks his head just right and contractions are strong.

However, sometimes it's clear that induction of labor is the best course of action. Your practitioner should review the pros and cons with you, in order for you to make an informed decision.

COMMON REASONS FOR LABOR INDUCTION

The most common reasons for inducing labor include:

- **Passing your due date.** Most practitioners will recommend induction if a pregnancy goes beyond 41 or 42 weeks.

- **Fetal stress or distress.** If there are concerns about the baby's well-being and you are near your due date, induction of labor may be the best choice. For babies farther from the due date, induction is used only when there is a serious concern about the baby's health in the uterus, and it is clearly better for the newborn to be cared for outside his mother's body.

- **Maternal illness.** Preeclampsia, uterine infection, or another medical condition may create a situation in which continuing the pregnancy may threaten the mother's health. Usually in these situations it is also better for the baby for birth to occur.

- **Premature rupture of the membranes.** If the bag of waters breaks before labor begins, the pros and cons of inducing labor will be assessed. Near full term, it is often better for the mother and baby if birth occurs sooner rather than later. If the bag of waters breaks early in the pregnancy, watchful waiting is often the better choice.

Your doctor has several options for inducing labor
Once the decision to induce has been made, your doctor will assess your condition and decide on the best way to proceed. In particular, she will determine the readiness of your cervix—that is, how dilated or effaced it already is. Here are some options:

- **Breaking the bag of waters.** If your cervix is already somewhat dilated and thinned out (or effaced), it may be enough for your practitioner to just break the amniotic sac, a procedure known as an amniotomy (see page 277). Many times, particularly in women who have had rapid labors in the past, this will give the uterus the chemical signals needed to start labor, and no further help is required.

- **Pitocin.** If your cervix is not quite so ready, or if the uterus does not respond to the breaking of the bag of waters, a medication called Pitocin can be used to get the uterus to contract. Pitocin is a synthetic version of oxytocin, the contraction-causing hormone naturally produced by a mother's own body. Usually, Pitocin is begun at a low dose and increased every 15 to 60 minutes until a normal labor pattern is reached. This means that you must have an IV and be continuously hooked up to a fetal monitor (see page 280) while you are on the medication. Often, an intrauterine pressure monitor, a thin tube that is inserted into the uterus next to the baby, is used to measure the strength of the contractions.

Pitocin inevitably makes the labor experience more high-tech and may preclude some anticipated comfort measures, such as standing in the shower, getting in the tub, or walking the halls. This may not be a problem for women using epidural anesthesia, but it can affect the coping power of a mom who desires natural childbirth. Women who are contemplating Pitocin and who desire natural childbirth should discuss the possibility of sitting in a rocking chair or walking around their room even if they need to be tethered to a monitor for the safety of the baby.

On the plus side, if the baby needs to be born because of a risk to the mom or baby, the ability to induce labor with Pitocin often prevents the medical staff from having to do a cesarean. In addition, in situations where the progress of active labor is slow (after a woman has reached four to five centimeters' dilation), the risk of cesarean is actually decreased if Pitocin is begun early, rather than waiting until labor has completely stalled. Some couples think of Pitocin as an unnecessary medical intervention, but if labor stalls, the drug actually may help them achieve their goal of a natural vaginal birth.

- **Medical agents for cervical ripening.** If the cervix is showing little sign of being ready, a so-called ripening agent (which makes the cervix softer, effaced, and slightly dilated) may be recommended before using Pitocin. The purpose of ripening the cervix before starting the contractions is to shorten the time needed for intense labor.

A good analogy is a child's party balloon: When you first start to blow into a balloon, it barely inflates at all, even if you blow very hard. However, once a certain size has been reached (about four centimeters), every breath makes a big difference. It's like that with contractions and cervices: Early on, lots of contractions are needed to get any dilation, but at a certain point (coincidentally, also at around four centimeters) the contractions make a bigger change.

The medications used to help ripen the cervix are all chemically related to the hormone prostaglandin E, which is naturally made by the body in other circumstances. It can take the form of a gel, tape, suppository, or tablet placed next to or inside the cervix, or it can be given orally.

- **Physical methods for cervical ripening.** Just as you might stretch out a balloon to make it easier to inflate, doctors will sometimes employ physical methods to ripen a cervix. One method involves inserting thin sticks of dried, sterilized seaweed (yes, really!) called laminaria or compressed foam into the cervix. Over the course of several hours, the sticks absorb moisture from the vagina and slowly expand, dilating the cervix. Another method is to insert a rubber balloon on the end of a tube (a Foley catheter) through the cervix. The balloon is inflated with water. Apparently, the pressure on the inside of the cervix gives the signal for dilation. Both of these methods also result in softening of the cervix.

Occasionally, using a cervical ripening technique prompts the uterus to contract, and labor ensues on its own. Most of the time, though, Pitocin is started 6 to 24 hours after treatment with the ripening agent is begun. Once labor is active, it usually progresses just like natural labor.

LOOKING AHEAD

On top of any anxiety or discomfort your little late-comer may have caused you, I have to warn you that post-date babies won't win any beauty contests—at least for a little while. An "overdue" baby may look as if he has been left in the bathtub too long. Aside from a set of wrinkles, he may have long fingernails and peeling skin. If meconium was present in the amniotic fluid, his skin even may have a slightly greenish cast. Don't worry. Post-date babies soon plump up and look as cute as the other babies. And some anecdotal evidence suggests that they actually may have a head start in the sleeping department. You deserve at least that much!

MYTHS ABOUT LABOR INDUCTION 🐝

Myth: Using Pitocin will cause the contractions to be too strong for the baby to handle.
Reality: When Pitocin is used to induce labor, both the baby's heartbeat and the timing of the uterine contractions are monitored carefully. If the baby's heart rate shows a worrisome pattern in response to the contractions, the dose of Pitocin is lowered. Sometimes the strength of the contractions is measured directly using an internal monitor (see page 282).

Myth: Contractions induced by Pitocin hurt more.
Reality: Some mothers have heard that contractions from Pitocin hurt more than natural labor. Of course, it is impossible to compare different experiences of labor, but most medical practitioners think that Pitocin-induced contractions mimic real ones—that is, in the beginning they are weaker and then grow more intense, and that overall they are comparable in strength. Why do women often report increased pain? For one thing, if a mom is having only weak contractions, the Pitocin certainly will make them stronger—after all, that's the whole point of administering it. Or perhaps the mother's mindset is different during an induction, or maybe she feels more uncomfortable because she's hooked up to a

monitor that prevents her from walking around. Perhaps the labor seems to take longer since all of it happens in the hospital. Or it could be that each time we labor, we are impressed anew at the intensity of the experience!

Myth: Induced labor will just end up requiring a cesarean section.
Reality: While most inductions result in the vaginal delivery of a healthy baby, there is, in fact, a higher chance of cesarean birth if induction is chosen. For this reason, induction usually is reserved for times when delivery by either means is clearly preferable to allowing the pregnancy to continue until labor starts naturally.

Myth: Induction of labor is a good way to allay fears about labor or to deliver on a schedule.
Reality: Some mothers wish that they could be induced because they are tired of being pregnant. Others have scheduling concerns, or worry that the baby will get too big for a vaginal delivery. There are indeed circumstances in which any of these might be a reason to induce labor, but the potential risks and benefits need to be carefully weighed.

NOTES

Use this space to jot down observations about your
pregnancy or questions to ask your healthcare practitioner at your next visit:

_____

_____

_____

_____

_____

_____

_____

_____

_____

_____

_____

_____

CHAPTER 11

Childbirth

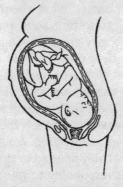

As her birthday dawns, your full-term baby is engaged deep in your pelvis. In preparation for labor, your cervix may have softened and shortened; powerful contractions of the uterine muscles will soon cause it to dilate, or open. When your cervix has dilated to 10 centimeters, you'll be able to push during contractions to help your baby into the world—and your waiting arms.

Throughout this book, we have talked about the development of your baby, signs of labor, the process of labor and birth, and common medical procedures. You have had a chance to think about what type of birth experience you would like and what and whom you want to have with you during labor. In this chapter, I'll discuss the remaining events of birth, as well as some key issues after the big day.

BEFORE BIRTH

OK, so you think you are in labor and you go to the hospital or birth center. What then? While routines vary from setting to setting, some practices are fairly universal. A nurse may greet you on arrival and settle you in. If it isn't clear that you're in active labor, you may go to a screening area, such as a medical exam room, where the baby's heart rate will be checked and your vital signs taken. The staff will ask if you've broken your water, when you last felt the baby move, and how often you are contracting. A fetal monitor (see page 280) will probably be used to check the baby and to see how she is responding to your contractions. An internal examination will probably be done. If you aren't yet in active labor, you may be asked to walk around for an hour or two before having another examination. During this time, have your coach stay with you. Once you are officially admitted to the hospital, you may get blood drawn and have an intravenous line started. This may not be necessary if you are planning on natural childbirth, but is needed if an epidural will be used. Some maternity units will place a heparin lock in your forearm or hand; this is a little capped-off IV line that can be used later if necessary to give fluids or medications. You won't find this confining: You can walk around and even shower with a "hep lock."

Breaking the bag of waters

Sometimes your amniotic sac, or bag of waters, breaks on its own before or during labor, and sometimes your practitioner makes a decision to assist this process. There are several reasons why it may be necessary for your doctor to perform an amniotomy, the intentional rupture of the membranes of the amniotic sac:

- **Labor induction.** Assisted rupture of membranes is sometimes used alone or in conjunction with medications to induce labor.
- **Labor augmentation.** An amniotomy can sometimes help labor progress more quickly. When a laboring mother's contractions are not as strong as they need to be, or labor is not progressing as fast as either the practitioner or the mother-to-be would like, this relatively simple procedure may be just the thing to help move the process along.
- **Access to the baby.** Babies may, on occasion, require internal monitoring (see page 282) during labor to watch the heartbeat more closely. Placing an internal monitor on a baby's scalp requires an opening in the bag of waters.
- **Checking for meconium.** When a mother-to-be gets close to delivering, her practitioner will often want to see if the baby has moved his bowels (or passed meconium—the first bowel movement) in the amniotic fluid (see page 282).

An amniotomy is usually done while the pregnant woman reclines with her legs bent at the knees and relaxed. In this position, the practitioner can most easily reach the vagina and the cervix. Usually this is no more painful than a vaginal exam. The practitioner uses a special sterile instrument called an amnio-hook, which resembles a plastic crochet hook, to make a hole in the amniotic sac. When it is torn, the amniotic fluid, in which the baby has been swimming for all these months, flows out. It is quite common to feel a warm sensation as the fluid leaves your body. Most women will continue to leak fluid until they deliver.

A baby's heart rate helps us know how he's handling labor

Babies were born for centuries without anyone check-ing their heart rates during labor. Now, whether you give birth at a hospital or a birth center, the staff is sure to assess your baby's heartbeat, either by listening peri-odically with a stethoscope—technically known as intermittent auscultation—or by using a fetal monitor. The heart rate tells us how the baby is handling labor's contractions. A normal fetal heart rate is between 120 and 160 beats per minute, although brief or minimal variations are common.

Intermittent auscultation isn't just random; it means listening to the baby's heart rate with a Doppler instrument or a fetal monitor at set times. Usually, this is done every 30 minutes in early labor, every 15 min-utes in active labor, and after every push or at least

BEFORE BIRTH   **279**

PARENT TO PARENT
"What do they do when they break your water? Does it hurt?"

—**Missy56482,** AS POSTED ON DRSPOCK.COM

"I've had my water broken all three times. They just take some sort of instrument and rupture the membrane. Does not hurt a bit."

—**momof3grls,** AS POSTED ON DRSPOCK.COM

"But I heard that it feels just like when the OB checks your cervix—you feel pressure. Is that true?"

—**Missy56482**

"Not for me. I didn't feel a thing, and I hadn't had my epidurals at that point. I had it done three times in order to get my labor going—and it did! My babies were born shortly afterward."

—**momof3grls**

every 5 minutes during the pushing phase. Generally, intermittent auscultation is a good choice for healthy mothers who have low-risk pregnancies. You can get into the shower or walk around, whatever works for you, which can be important as you try to remain comfortable in the later phases of labor. Intermittent auscultation also may give you a more natural birth experience, since you are not constantly connected to machines.

There are no risks to intermittent auscultation as long as everything is going well. Research has shown that babies watched with this sort of low-tech assessment do just as well as ones who are continuously hooked up to a fetal monitor. In fact, the one surprising research finding was that intermittent auscultation appeared to actually *decrease* the chance of having a cesarean: Continuous heart-rate monitoring (that is, being constantly hooked up to a fetal monitor) sometimes shows abnormalities that turn out to be false alarms, leading to, in retrospect, unnecessary cesarean sections.

Fetal monitors provide more extensive information

Often, when you arrive at the hospital, your health-care team may hook you up to an external fetal monitor for 20 minutes. This machine, which measures both your baby's heart rate and the timing and length of your contractions, gives the team an initial assessment of how well the baby is tolerating labor. If the heart rate is within the normal range, shows good variability (fluctuations), and provides no evidence of worrisome slowing, it is said to be reassuring, meaning that the baby seems to be in good condition. In that case, your practitioner may continue to monitor your labor electronically, or take off the monitor and simply check the baby's heart rate at regular intervals (the intermittent auscultation I just mentioned).

If the baby is at risk for fetal distress due to an abnormal heart-rate pattern, maternal medical problems such as high blood pressure, or use of medications such as Pitocin or epidural anesthesia, continuous electronic monitoring is usually recommended. And if an external monitor isn't giving adequate information, internal contraction monitoring (see page 282) or internal fetal heart-rate monitoring may be recommended. The latter uses a thin wire attached to the scalp to transmit electrical signals from your baby's heart, allowing the heartbeat to be followed moment by moment.

It's pretty common for the fetal heart rate to go through a phase that looks a bit worrisome. If the healthcare team detects a potential problem, you may be asked to change positions (usually shifting to your left side). This can relieve compression on the umbilical cord or on the blood flow to your uterus. In addition, you may be given oxygen for a short time and extra fluid through an intravenous (IV) line. Often these simple actions are all that is needed to make the baby appear stable and healthy once again. If there is a sign of a serious problem, steps may be taken to deliver the baby quickly by cesarean section.

If continuous fetal monitoring is recommended, most moms-to-be typically stay in bed. The cords from the monitor reach about eight feet, so sometimes you can pace around near the monitor or sit in a rocker at the bedside. Some childbirth centers have portable telemetry units, which attach in the same way as a standard monitor but transmit the signal to a base unit without cords, like a portable phone. Telemetry allows the mother who requires continuous monitoring to walk around during labor.

An intrauterine-pressure catheter monitors contractions closely

Particularly if labor is being induced with Pitocin (see page 268) or progressing slowly, your practitioner may want to keep careful track of your contractions. Usually, the hospital staff starts by using an external contraction monitor, but while this device indicates the timing of the contractions, it doesn't accurately measure their intensity. When a more complete picture of the contractions is needed, your practitioner may recommend internal contraction monitoring with an intrauterine-pressure catheter (IUPC).

The IUPC, which is usually used in combination with fetal heart-rate monitoring, measures the actual pressure within the uterus and indicates the frequency and intensity of contractions. A thin, flexible tube with a small pressure-sensing device on the tip is inserted into the uterus next to the baby. The IUPC can be inserted if the cervix is at least a little dilated, and once the water has broken.

The IUPC also can be used for amnio-infusion, the infusion of sterile fluid into the uterus. This can be helpful if an infant has had a bowel movement before birth, which is known as meconium staining of the amniotic fluid. Usually, amniotic fluid is clear or straw-colored. If the fluid appears yellow or green, the baby may have passed her first bowel movement, known as meconium. Meconium sometimes is passed when a fetus is in distress, but most of the time its presence is just a sign that the baby's intestinal tract is maturing as she approaches full term. At birth, if meconium is present in the fluid, your practitioner will suction out the baby's nose and mouth just after her head comes out, so she won't inhale the meconium particles with her first breath. Amnio-infusion also can be used to dilute the amniotic fluid and consequently decrease the likelihood that the baby will suffer complications from inhaling thick, meconium-stained fluid at birth.

Sometimes there is evidence of compression of the umbilical cord during labor, leading to slowing of the fetal heart rate. Amnio-infusion may help cushion the cord and diminish the stress on the baby. Your healthcare team will make recommendations if this is indicated.

DURING BIRTH

So you have gone through labor, whether short or long, mild or intense, and have reached complete dilation. When you reach the point of pushing, you may actually feel a sense of relief that the time has finally come and you are able to play an active role in this part of child-

Q: Do I have to have internal monitoring?

A: Childbirth is a natural process, and you may be thinking that electrodes and other monitoring devices are as far from natural as could be. If you have a question about whether or not any particular procedure is necessary, feel free to ask your practitioner. Most women in labor don't require more than a check on the fetal heartbeat at regular intervals. Your preferences can be taken into account, especially in nonemergency circumstances. And while using these monitors may not be your image of the perfect labor, if they become necessary, do keep in mind that you and your practitioner have common goals: a healthy baby and a healthy mother!

birth. Fatigued as you are, you may discover a new-found energy and enthusiasm for pushing. You may feel intense rectal pressure or as if you need to have a bowel movement. You also may experience a stretching or burning sensation, as pressure on the vaginal opening (perineum) is increased. You may start trembling and feel a tremendous sense of excitement.

To push effectively, you must find a comfortable position

You might push in several different positions before you actually give birth. In most of the pushing positions, you should think of rounding your body into a C position, tucking your chin into your chest and rounding your back. Your coaches can help support you in this position. It is helpful to grasp your thighs behind your knees, for extra leverage, as you round into your C position.

Pushing is easier if gravity is helping you. Squatting or kneeling lets you push with gravity in your favor. Sometimes, if the baby is having difficulty getting under the pubic bone, lying on your back with your legs flexed back (thighs brought up toward your chest) can be very effective. You may also want to get on your hands and knees to push. It is often a good idea to change positions numerous times during pushing, to see which works best for you and your baby.

Breathing techniques also help you push effectively as well as relax between contractions. There are several ways to breathe as you push. Much of this will be dictated by which method of childbirth education you are using and what feels right. The important thing to remember is to take your cleansing breaths, get into position, and use your breathing technique until the end of the contraction. Rest between contractions as much as possible. Close your eyes. Try to relax all your muscles as you breathe out. Some women don't want any physical contact right now, but if you find your partner's touch soothing, ask him for a gentle leg massage in between contractions; it can feel absolutely wonderful after the hard work of pushing.

When you feel a contraction starting to build, bear down as if you were having a bowel movement. Keep the push at a constant pressure. Relax your bottom as much as possible as you bear down. It may be helpful to have a warm washcloth on your perineum, to relax the muscles and to help you focus on pushing toward that area. You may also want to have the nurse or doula bring in a mirror so that you can see the opening of the birth canal as you bear down. Seeing the top of your baby's head as you push can give you the encouragement you need to keep going.

As your baby's head appears (or crowns), you may feel stinging and stretching at the opening of your vagina.

PARENT TO PARENT
"I'm one of the lucky moms who get to tell their birth stories without scaring people! In my first pregnancy, I went into labor five days early (with no false labor to fake me out beforehand). The first several hours weren't too bad; my husband and I went to buy a CD player and rented a movie to watch in the hospital (Jerry McGuire—everyone always wants to know). My contractions had slowed down by this time, so we went home and I took a shower. Then the contractions speeded up and began

Your obstetrician may do an episiotomy (see page 288) if it seems necessary. After your practitioner delivers the baby's head, she may ask you not to push as she suctions the baby's nose and mouth. She will tell you when to push again to deliver the baby's body. As you push the baby out, remember to open your eyes and experience this miracle fully. You are seeing the top of the head that you will kiss a million times, that you will love in a way that is hard to describe. Appreciate the moment!

to really hurt. We decided to go to the hospital then, not so much because we thought I'd made much progress, but because I was starting to feel nauseous, and I figured if I was going to throw up, I might as well have someone else clean it up! When we got to Labor & Delivery, the nurse told me I was dilated five centimeters. My water broke during the next contraction, and five contractions later, my baby's head was half out (I kid you not—no pushing involved). There! Is that a good birth story for you?"

—coloradomom, AS POSTED ON DRSPOCK.COM

The afterbirth comes next

In the excitement of the birth of your baby, you may forget about the placenta, but your doctor or midwife will still need to deliver it. After your baby is born, the placenta will separate from the wall of the uterus. As this occurs, you may feel an urge to push, or your practitioner may tell you to bear down, and the placenta will be delivered. Don't be afraid of this one last push; the placenta is much smaller and more flexible than the baby was. After it is expelled, most moms feel a great sense of relief and realize that their stomachs are noticeably flatter.

Your practitioner will examine your placenta to make sure it is intact and no fragments are left inside your uterus. You may want to see it. Note the maternal and fetal sides, the umbilical cord attachment, and the blood vessels. The placenta sustained your baby's life while inside you. It is a fascinating component of the miracle of birth.

Some doctors are fonder of episiotomies than others

An episiotomy is a surgical incision at the opening of the vagina. Its purpose is to allow more room for delivery and to prevent tears of the tissues around the vagina. Some practitioners believe that an episiotomy protects the pelvic muscles and helps the woman maintain normal function of those muscles later in her life. Others believe it causes damage to the vaginal opening and surrounding muscles. These conflicting beliefs help to explain why there are different rates of episiotomy with different practitioners, birth settings, and cultures.

Some practitioners perform an episiotomy on all first-time mothers, but many wait to see if it seems necessary. In a first pregnancy, it is hard to say for sure if an episiotomy will be required until the baby's head has applied pressure to the vaginal opening (perineum) for a while. Some perineums are stretchier than others.

Whether or not to perform an episiotomy is a judgment call. If you are expecting a very large baby, the practitioner might do an episiotomy to make delivery easier. If delivery is needed quickly, as in the case of fetal distress, the vaginal opening doesn't have time to stretch, and an episiotomy may be required. If, after multiple pushes, all that stands between you and your baby is persistently tight skin, or if the tissues up at the front of the vagina are beginning to tear, most practitioners will do one.

Sometimes, without an episiotomy, multiple tears can occur, and the process of sewing them up is worse for the mother than if a single incision were done. In my practice, about half of first-time mothers get an episiotomy. Even if you require an episiotomy with your first birth, the chance of needing one during subsequent deliveries is lower.

While some practitioners say that recovery's easier from a laceration than from an episiotomy, either one can be quite uncomfortable for a week or more. Ice packs are helpful for the first 24 hours, and hot soaks in sitz baths after that. Witch-hazel pads (such as Tucks) and anesthetic spray are often offered in the hospital, and can be continued at home. A doughnut-shaped inflatable pillow, available from the hospital or your local drugstore, can make sitting more comfortable. The stitches dissolve on their own. While it is not uncommon to have some discomfort for many weeks after birth, most practitioners want to know if you are still having pain at six weeks.

Forceps and vacuum-assisted births can help ensure vaginal delivery

Occasionally, a woman needs a little help from her practitioner to complete a vaginal delivery. Your doctor

---

PREVENTING EPISIOTOMIES

There are exercises to do in the third trimester that may help prevent lacerations or the need for episiotomy at delivery. These involve stretching the vaginal opening with a technique called perineal massage. You or your partner can gently put two or more fingers about two to three inches into your vagina and press down and out on the vaginal opening.

Most pregnant women find that, if doing perineal massage themselves, they need to use the thumbs of each hand in order to reach. Stretch to the point of mild discomfort and hold it for a few minutes. Consciously relax the muscles as you massage. Using a lubricant like K-Y jelly or mineral oil may make it more comfortable. Repeat this exercise as often as every day in the third trimester.

may need to pull gently on the baby's head while you push. The use of vacuum or forceps to assist in delivery is referred to as assisted or operative vaginal delivery. Operative vaginal delivery can only be done if the baby has free access to the birth canal—meaning that the cervix is fully dilated and the baby is expected to fit through without a problem.

In some cases, a baby needs to be delivered more quickly than a mother could reasonably be expected to push him out. Usually this is because the baby has a

The theory is that perineal massage can imitate the stretching process of birth and get the vagina ready, since a woman is much less likely to tear or need an episiotomy after she has given birth once. It is unclear if perineal massage really does help prevent lacerations, since research in this area is scanty. Many well-intentioned couples find the exercises annoying or uncomfortable to do, and quit before it could be expected to be helpful.

During childbirth, warm compresses on the perineum during the pushing stage can help with discomfort but probably won't protect you from needing an episiotomy or tearing. Perineal massage during the pushing stage, with mineral oil or other lubricant, may be helpful. The best protection is a slow, controlled birth, with a practitioner experienced in avoiding lacerations and episiotomies.

slow heartbeat. Another common reason for operative vaginal delivery is when the mother has been pushing for a long time and is getting exhausted. If a little extra power will make the difference, assisted vaginal delivery is an option. In cases where the cervix is not adequately dilated, a cesarean section is usually needed.

Forceps are smooth metal instruments, shaped like long, narrow spoons, that are carefully applied to the sides of the baby's head. As the mother bears down, the doctor will guide the baby's head. When the head is partway out, the forceps are slipped off, one at a time, and the mother is usually encouraged to complete the delivery on her own.

A vacuum extractor is used for the same purpose. In this case, a plastic cup is placed on the baby's head and attached to a suction device. Again, the baby moves down the birth canal using both sources of power, the mother's pushing and the pulling of the vacuum.

Each method has slightly different advantages, disadvantages, and risks. Both have been shown, in scientific studies, to be safe and effective when properly used. There are some drawbacks, though: There may be temporary red marks on the baby's cheeks from the forceps, or a bruise on the top of the head if vacuum is used; the marks usually fade in a few days. In addition, both methods increase the chance that the mother's vagina may tear or that an episiotomy will be needed. (However, many moms prefer this possibility to the certainty of a surgical incision from a cesarean.) Each practitioner has an opinion about which instrument will be more useful in a particular situation. If you have a strong preference, bring this up with your practitioner during your prenatal office visits.

AFTER BIRTH

When your baby is born she will be wet with amniotic fluid, and may be covered by a sticky, creamy substance called vernix, which is a lot like lanolin. Her head may be slightly elongated (the shape helped her fit through the birth canal). It will look more rounded in a few days.

Many hospitals have routine procedures for newborns. The timing of the procedures will depend upon your hospital's protocols, the course of your labor, the condition of your baby at birth, and your preferences.

Immediately after birth:

- After the baby's head comes out, your practitioner may clean out the baby's nose and mouth with a suction bulb.

- After the rest of the baby is delivered, either your practitioner or your support person will cut the umbilical cord.

- At your request, the birth team may immediately place your baby on your chest to start the bonding process. Your baby can be dried off, kept warm, and assessed while he is with you. This is really great if you can arrange it—it is wonderful to have your baby near you right from the start.

- At one minute after birth, the pediatrician or labor nurse will assign your baby an Apgar score (see box below). This score helps the medical team decide if he needs oxygen or other forms of medical support. Another Apgar score will be given at five minutes.

THE MEANING OF THE APGAR SCORE 🐎

As soon as your baby makes her way into this world, doctors or nurses will be assessing the basics: her activity, heart rate, and breathing. They will give her a numerical score at one minute and again at five minutes. These scores help the medical team assess how much (if any) medical help the baby needs in the first few minutes of life.

Developed by an anesthesiologist named Dr. Virginia Apgar, this test rates the baby 0, 1, or 2 points on each of five newborn characteristics:

- heart rate
- breathing
- muscle tone
- reflexes
- skin color.

An Apgar score of 7 or better signifies that the baby is in good condition. If the baby rates between 4 and 6 at the one-minute Apgar, she will usually need some

- It is very important to keep newborns warm. Your baby will be wrapped in blankets, or, if you want, you can place him next to your skin and lay blankets over the two of you.

---

help. Oxygen will be administered, and she may have her airway suctioned. Those babies who score under 4 need more extraordinary measures of resuscitation. Narcotic medications, given to the mother for pain relief in labor, can contribute to a lower score.

Most of the time, if the Apgar score is low at one minute, by five minutes it's back to 7 or higher. If this is the case, the low one-minute score really means nothing; the baby will do fine. If the Apgar score is still under 7 after the second assessment, another score is usually assigned at 10 minutes. If it comes up to 7 or above by then, again, the baby will probably do well. Only if the Apgar score stays quite low for more than 10 minutes is there a high likelihood of a real problem.

Many parents worry that their baby may not be OK if the Apgar score is low. Don't panic. The first 10 minutes of life is a very resilient time for babies. Even those who have difficulties in this period generally do well. Pediatricians know that the Apgar score has no bearing at all on a child's future SAT scores, personality, learning, or anything else.

- This is your chance to meet the being who's been moving and kicking inside you all these months. You can hold him close, look into his eyes, and start getting to know your little one. You may notice that the baby is making movements with his mouth when he wants to feed. If you have chosen to breastfeed, this would be an ideal time to nurse your baby. This is also a nice time to take some early pictures.

- If a surgical clamp was used on the umbilical cord, it will be switched for a small plastic clip, similar in appearance to a hair barrette. A few weeks later, the dried-up cord stump will fall off.

Within the first hour after birth:

- The nurse or doctor will examine your baby and check her vital signs.

- She will be weighed, and her length and head circumference will be measured. This is always a nice photo opportunity, if your partner or another visitor wants to take some pictures that show the weight on the scale.

- Identification bands will be placed on your baby's wrist and ankle. You will receive an ID band that matches her bands. The nurse may record your infant's footprints.

- State laws require that your baby's eyes be treated with an antibiotic within one hour of birth to prevent blindness from maternal vaginal infections. Most hospitals use erythromycin ointment.

- Your baby will receive an injection of vitamin K in her thigh. This vitamin is important for blood clotting. In an adult, bacteria in the intestines manufacture vitamin K. Newborns have no bacteria in their intestines; consequently, they are not able to produce vitamin K on their own.

- A blood sugar test may be necessary if your baby is very large or very small, or if you had gestational diabetes (see page 147). Usually the baby's heel is pricked to get a drop of blood. If the baby's blood sugar (glucose) is too low, you may be asked to nurse your baby or give her some formula or sugar water.

If you are worried about your baby, or think that you heard something about the events during or after birth that puts your baby at risk, talk to your doctor. Many parents have worried needlessly due to misunderstandings about the events of labor and delivery.

Postpartum depressed feelings, fatigue, and other emotional changes
The first few days after the baby is born can be very intense. You may be exhausted from labor or exhilarated about the baby's arrival—or both. You may have a private room or share your room with another new mother. If you have your own room, it may be possible for the baby's father to stay with you as you get to know your newborn. If you have other children at home, of course, this may not be possible. On average, a hospital stay consists of two nights after a vaginal birth and three after a cesarean.

It is vital to take care of yourself during the postpartum period, particularly the first two to four weeks after the baby comes home. Over these weeks, if you find yourself totally exhausted or you begin to feel panicky, call your spouse or partner, a healthcare practitioner, a friend, or anyone who can offer you support. It is important to realize that there is a close relationship between postpartum exhaustion and emotional overload. On the other hand, being tearful can be totally normal. Even when everything goes well, you may feel very emotional, particularly starting two or three days after the baby is born. This is called the baby blues and happens to about 70 percent of new mothers throughout the world. The blues are probably caused by changes in the levels of the pregnancy hormones after delivery, but their exact cause is unknown. Have confidence that the feelings will pass—perhaps within days, perhaps within a few weeks. Most mothers with the baby blues know deep down that nothing is really wrong. This emotional state goes away on its own.

If your mood interferes with daily activities or lasts more than a few weeks, you may be experiencing something more severe than the blues. Postpartum depression affects 10 to 15 percent of new mothers and can include feelings of hopelessness and anxiety. Women with a history of depression or a family history of mental health problems are more likely to have emotional difficulties postpartum. Troubling thoughts can keep coming into the mind of the new mother. Women sometimes feel that they don't love their new baby, and some even feel like harming the baby or themselves. Some women have difficulty sleeping, while others feel like sleeping all the time. The worst part is that the new mom becomes convinced that these feelings are inevitable and that she will never feel like herself again.

It's important to know that postpartum depression is treatable, but you will need the help of a trained professional, and you may require medication. Many medications are safe for breastfeeding babies, and since you are the most important person in the world to your newborn, it is important that you take good care of yourself. Don't let postpartum emotional difficulties make a time that should be full of joy into a nightmare for you and your family—seek out the help you need.

Taking your new baby home

Taking a first baby home from the hospital or birth center can be a very odd feeling. I remember that my husband and I looked at each other and said, "*Now* what do we do?" It will take days or even weeks until you get into a routine. During this time, it is a good idea, as much as possible, to have two adults around most of the time. Being alone with a newborn can be overwhelming.

The secret of survival during this time is low expectations: Set realistic goals, like getting the baby fed and changed as often as necessary, and trying to eat, sleep, and shower when you need to. Notice that the list does not include preparing meals, cleaning the house, or entertaining guests! As much as possible, limit guests to people who will really help you—not those you may feel a need to entertain.

If friends or relatives ask what they can do to help, here are some ideas: Have them watch the baby while you take a shower. Ask them to bring over a meal. Suggest that they do some laundry, wash the dishes, empty the dishwasher, or clean up the kitchen. You may feel as if you're imposing, but people really do want to be helpful at a time like this. And don't be shy about telling your partner what you need. For example, maybe he could bring you the baby at night to nurse in bed, order and pick up some take-out food, or do a load of laundry. If it's financially feasible, you might consider hiring a baby nurse or a postpartum doula to provide a little professional assistance.

Bringing a baby home is an awesome, life-changing responsibility, but you will be surprised how much will come naturally to you and your partner. As Dr. Benjamin Spock wrote in his venerable *Baby and Child Care*, "Trust yourself. You know more than you think you do." That's what my husband and I discovered when we brought our son home from the hospital. And that's what you're sure to discover too. So, congratulations, Mom and Dad, and thank you for letting me come along with you on your amazing journey to parenthood.

NOTES

Use this space to jot down observations or questions to ask your healthcare practitioner at your next visit:

_____

_____

_____

_____

_____

_____

_____

_____

_____

_____

_____

_____

_____

INDEX